Mary, Mary Nurse Contrai

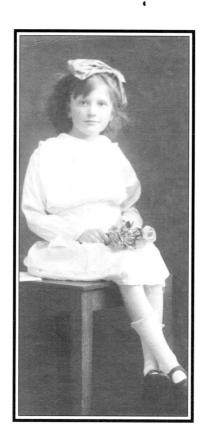

The life of
Mary Alicia Hodkinson
1912 - 1995

by Anne Bradley

Foreword

Mary Hodkinson was a remarkable person. Her dedicated service to the community had given her insights into life which few ever achieve. Time spent with her always included very interesting conversation, illustrated with fascinating stories of her experiences.

In her later life, Mary Hodkinson discovered that higher education could provide a supportive environment to take forward her own enjoyment of learning but also an opportunity for her to serve and support the needs of her fellow older learners. She established Life Long Learning as a significant activity within the University of Central Lancashire by demonstrating what could be achieved if there was determination to succeed. Each time we met she had progress and new directions to report on the wide range of projects in which she was involved.

Even when she became too ill to join in activities at the University, visits to her home were still characterised by discussions about the future and what she wanted to achieve.

Mary Hodkinson is remembered by the wider University community in many different ways and in a special corner there is a small acknowledgement of the very significant contribution she made to the University.

This book reflects the diversity and richness of experience which was the life of Mary Hodkinson.

It was my privilege to know Mary Hodkinson in the latter years of her life.

Brian Booth, *Vice-Chancellor*
University of Central Lancashire
November 1997

Acknowledgements

The staff of the Lancashire Library; the Lancashire Records Office; the Lancashire Evening Post Library; the University of Central Lancashire, Preston; The Records Department, Queen Mary's Hospital, Carshalton; Maritime Museum, Liverpool;

The Arts and Libraries Officer, Kent County Council.

The staff of The Willows Child Development and Family Support Centre, Ashton, Preston.

The Headteachers of Deepdale Infant and Junior Schools.

St. Catherine's Hospice, Lostock Hall, Bamber Bridge. • The Nurses' League, Preston.

Rev. Dennis Duckworth, Swedenborgian Minister, Whetstone, London.

Jersey Evening Post • Mr. E. & Mr. F. Steele, Fulwood, Preston.

Mr. & Mrs. J. C. Best. • Miss Florence Chew.

Mrs Catherine Duckworth • Mrs. Joyce Ramsbottom.

For photographs.

Mr. Arthur Hodgson. • Mrs. W. T. Singleton. • The Reference Library, Birmingham City Libraries.
Knight, Frank & Rutley, Tunbridge Wells, Kent. • Nursing Mirror.

For typing and computer processing and use of family records
Miss Margaret Hodkinson
With thanks for unflagging co-operation

Contents

Contents

Introduction

I was well into scribbling Mary's spoken recollections of her early days before I knew there had been such a person as Elise for whom she had assumed total responsibility, not only in the small worker's cottage where we were sitting, but over a period of 46 years.

If a posy of flowers was brought by a friend they were placed in a vase, as an offering, near to the one picture that existed of this lady older than Mary, taken by a photographer in a London street during the 1951 Exhibition. Mary's loyalty to the memory of her emotionally damaged and memory-impaired ex- colleague, was total.

I have noticed that those who care, in their personal lives, voluntarily and unremittingly for a handicapped person have 'something extra', as though, having demanded so much from themselves, they expect nothing from others - there is enough to go round, a space filled with patience and acceptance.

There I sat, supposed to be recording the notable incidents of a varied life of achievement, particularly in the field of nursing the elderly sick, yet, what was most remarkable was passed over, mentioned as incidental when it affected the action: a total nursing commitment to one who was not a relative, or, even in the true sense of the word, a friend.

Not only was there the mystery of Elise's identity but, to me the mystery of utter confidence expressed in Mary's life - and on the brink of death - that all would be well. Who was the Trustee? I had met women of high administrative ability before and they had, even in old age, this driving quality in common: "I could do it and you can do it," countenancing no refusal to facilitate that creative energy whose expression leads to drawing things spontaneously together and making them work in social harmony.

So here is the story as the facts fell from Mary's lips, with clear selective recall, beginning in the Wigan shop where her father died. She had retained files of documentation from her nursing life and she knew that if she were to die (which she was striving not to do) before all was recalled, that I had these records. She had begun to sort them when the doctor had given the ultimatum.

It is characteristic of the reaction to Mary's unconforming spirit that these written words should excite opposing attitudes. One young specialist nurse with whom I verified some described nursing procedures said. "She was a whirlwind - she would have had a very high-powered job these days." But do persons of total honesty and forthrightness reach that sort of power?

Mary did not seek out well-known hospitals or nursing homes of high repute. She went where need was great and one can envisage her, had she lived at the century's end working in the field with aid agencies.

A comment has been made that full professional achievement came late and that there was no overall plan. One answer to that is: unless one had experienced the responsibility it is difficult to conceive the irrelevance to the war effort of any chronic civilian illness, least of all such a one from which Elise suffered.

The wonder is that Mary could, during the stringencies that prevailed, support her handicapped colleague in working mode for so long. Without Mary hers would have been a discarded life. And, a unity there was: from Mary's teen-age care of her grandmother to her spearheading the movement for geriatric care.

Did the pain control treatment of her cancer affect Mary's sharpness of mind? I, nor any other person observed any haziness, any loss of clarity. To the end there was that high self trust, an instinct that confounds criticism.

All this happened to Mary from a world tour by sea during the 1914-1918 Great War; to a Workhouse Hospital; to medically assisting Freedom Fighters in World War 11; to upsetting the Government in an offshore island after the war; to her appointing to replace herself the first male Matron in the country; to instigating a Geriatric Care Association which fostered enthusiasm and knowledge for <u>all</u> workers in this field and gave tremendous feed-back to put pressure on powerful decision makers. Even her idealistic vision of a Geriatric Centre has in modified local forms, come about.

She was a nettle in the side of entrenched middle management, but her ideas did reach the top where action was taken. Betty, wife of Rev. J. C. Best, herself a very experienced community nurse expressed her own view " Florence Nightingale was the first trouble shooter in nursing, I reckon Mary was a close second."

In her own old age, even whilst caring for her sick dependent, Mary's social hobby was prodding people to be inquisitive, to take a walk, to support each other in all pleasant activities. The little quarterly magazine *Life Long Learning News*, which her sister Margaret now edits and sees through to press under the auspices of the University of Central Lancashire at Preston is her lively baby.

I hope she will, with this true story, prod the reader as she prodded me.

Anne Bradley, Higher Walton, January 1997.

From Wigan to World Tour

The medical details of her arrival into the world on 18th September 1912 fascinated Mary Alicia. She could not ignore the marks of the forceps on her forehead noticeable until early middle life. A grave decision had been made, too, as her mother had been given chloroform and there was no way of knowing if the patient was allergic to it. It was a Wednesday.

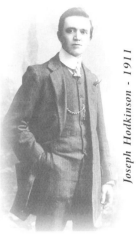

Joseph Hodkinson - 1911

Her father was Joseph Hodkinson, one of a family of 13 who were members of the New Jerusalem Church (Swedenborgian) in Wigan. Joseph was a lay preacher and when he visited Preston to preach, he met Miss Edith Mary Clarkson who, like Joseph, was a member of a family who had been Swedenborgians for four generations. She was a milliner, working in a haberdasher's shop in town. They continued a mode of courtesy by which a person was addressed and spoken of by title 'Mr. Mrs. etc'. They became engaged to be married after an acquaintance of twelve months during which due to their advanced age (27 and 30) a chaperone was not obligatory. Money was not discussed - this being bad form - but Miss Clarkson had a certain prudence so consulted a local person with an Ouija board and asked "what does Joseph Hodkinson earn?" The answer spelled out the word 'Money'. Edith married him, bore and brought up three children who treated the anecdote with hilarity.

Their first child Mary was born in King Street, Wigan but not long

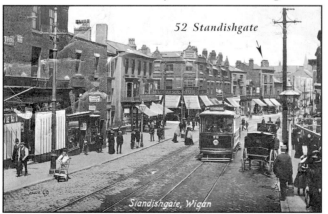

after Joseph was established enough in his watchmaker's and jeweller's business to move to 52 Standishgate. The adjoining shop, a florist's, needed only the ground floor so Joseph had the use of all the cellars, also the

52 Standishgate

Postcard to Grandparents' Clarkson - 1913

first and second floor rooms above both shops. The upstairs drawing room was so large that he planned to install a full size church organ in the chimney alcove. Two suites were upholstered in blue velvet, the three-seater sofas would convert into chaises longues. Here were held musical soirees with other business and professional people as guests. There was a resident maid and a daily woman for rough work.

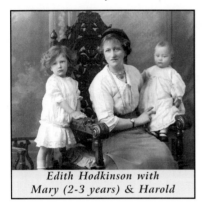

Edith Hodkinson with Mary (2-3 years) & Harold

A bright future was planned for the young first-born. Father decided she was to be an interior designer and he built her a big dolls' house on the second floor and she was to have free range to furnish. Many years later Mary did have scope in her career for interior design, but it was re-arranging furniture in geriatric hospitals.

Only 13 months after Mary, brother Harold was born and before Mary was five a third baby, Margaret. The busy mother, who was also learning to do the business accounts was glad to let Mary spend much of her time in the shop downstairs away from the new baby and from young Harold whose good health was not yet established.

Mary loved the peace in the shop and liked to conceal herself behind the fixtures. Her favourite hiding place was behind the aspidistra in a jardiniere poised on a mahogany column. Customers received a shock when entering an apparently empty shop a childish voice, well instructed in formal courtesy, piped: "Forward, Mr. Hodkinson, please" and her father materialised from his workshop.

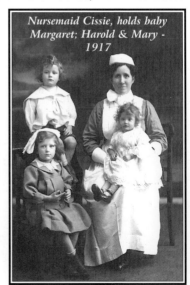

Nursemaid Cissie, holds baby Margaret; Harold & Mary - 1917

The maid Cissie escorted Mary to her first school, a small private establishment in a Standishgate house. When Mary was collected at midday, she was standing on the steps to the street holding out her hand to the teacher saying "Thank you very much for having me. I shall not be coming any more. Your children are too rough and noisy". The long quiet hours spent with her father had a profound effect on Mary, a lasting appreciation of peace and silent companionship.

This warm relationship with her father was rudely shattered: within six weeks of Mary's first half day at school Joseph was dead and Mary was not at school again until she had completed a world tour. Her father was a victim albeit in undramatic circumstances of the First World War.

By 1917 there had been three years of carnage on the battlefields of France. Conscription required age groups -late 30's- to attend for medical examination. Stripped and waiting in a draughty hut, Joseph developed pleurisy. Partially recovered after hospitalisation he was sent to a convalescent home at Grange-over-Sands. He returned home from there seeming well enough and played the piano at Mary's birthday party. She was five when her father died, officially from pneumonia, on the 15th October 1917,

The two older children were taken to the neat bedroom as he lay there and told that Daddy had gone to sleep and would not wake up. He was going to stay with Jesus who needed him. They would not see him any more but he would always be near them. Harold, nearly four years old, timid and sickly, took his Mother's hand and said "Don't worry Mother, I'll be Father now".

Later that day Mary was taken outdoors under a clear autumn sky. One star twinkled brightly. Her mother said this was "Daddy's Star" and a sign that he was always thinking of them. It was a simple belief that sustained Mary in the trials to come.

Brother and sister attended the funeral service at the New Jerusalem Church in Wigan. Each carried a Madonna lily whose white trumpet flower erect on the stem was taller than they were.

Mr. Hodkinson had been a popular business man and local memories also lingered on of his father, an enlightened coal mine owner who, after a serious mine flood, had installed pumping gear and was able to keep men employed for another 14 years.

As the cortege moved along Standishgate it was lined with people paying their last respects to a courteous man of business, the official clock winder and repairer for the Borough and a notable lay preacher.

Financially the family was ruined. As an apparently strong young man Joseph had acted confidently with his trade, investing wisely in equipment to expand his business. He had paid cash to purchase gold and silver plating baths and had handed over money to colleagues who were planning similar ventures. Unusually he had not obtained receipts but had acted on the old understanding that a gentleman's word is his bond.

Sales apart from watch repairs for soldiers had fallen drastically during the war years. Joseph's widow never recovered any money. Worse was revealed. To assemble the cash Joseph had let his life insurance payments lapse.

However, the possibility of his wife becoming a war-widow had been faced and a plan suggested. Edith Mary Hodkinson, rigorously conscientious to her spoken word, had agreed and now intended to fulfil it.

At the time of his marriage in 1911 her husband had financed the passage to Australia of three of his sisters. His wife had no sisters, though five brothers. It was a fond assumption that the fatherless children would be assisted to a better life by their aunts in Australia. So, to find the means to travel there, the business must be sold. Furniture, silver, china, jewellery was auctioned. After the purchase of second-class tickets for £90 for one adult and three children there was £48 left. Unsold silver and jewellery was packed to be later sold for living expenses and as gifts for relatives. Further confidence was given by a letter of introduction to the Australian agent of the Preston printing business in which the children's Uncle Jack was engaged.

Mary's beautiful dolls' house, so large that she could walk into it, was converted into packing cases. The tickets for sailing were late arriving but, with his usual thoroughness, Uncle Jack got things moving. Later he wished he had allowed the muddle to reign, as he knew that his sister would have called off the whole expedition which he deplored from the start.

The U-boat blockade had been all too successful. On the 31st January 1918 when the family were aboard the Ionic it was the last sailing of women and children for Australia during the War.

Uncle Jack had arranged for identity tags for the children to be printed on waterproof material. Three to four inches wide and two inches long they were firmly sewn on to the inside of their vests: 'To whom it may concern: if this child should be picked up alive OR dead in the Northern Hemisphere contact John Clarkson (address): in the Southern Hemisphere contact Mary Hodkinson (Australian address of Aunt). The care of this child will be rewarded'. Mary was very proud of this proof of her own worth alive or dead and managed to keep it, transferred to other vests, on dry land, until she was nearly eight years old.

At five years old sailing to Australia, like the other passengers, she was required to wear a life-belt at all times, and near the war zone, had to go to bed fully clothed even to an overcoat with a cork life belt on top.

Measles rather than U-boats was the menace on the six weeks sail. All the afflicted child passengers were carried from individual cabins to the big comfortable sofas in the lounges. Mary had her jointed doll which her father had given her when she was two, a beloved toy which she kept for 60 years before giving it to an orphaned child. Baby Margaret, 15 months old, who had ceased to talk or walk after her father died, was poorly as well. Mrs. Hodkinson kept a log of the practicalities of the entire trip, written between her bedside ministrations with games and books. It became a family keepsake.

The family was received at Kilda, a suburb of Sydney where the three children, lively by this time, disrupted the Aunts' quiet life, especially during the preparations for Aunt Mary's April wedding.

The remnants of silver and jewellery now given as presents, made the newcomers appear affluent. But the future looked bleak. A policy of equal pay for equal work, made paying for child care out of reach if Mrs. Hodkinson were to find work. Welcome in the family was cool and Edith was having second thoughts about the whole venture.

She sought advice from Uncle Jack's Sydney agent with the letter she had brought. Her brother Jack together with the owners of the *Lancashire Daily Post*, the Toulmin brothers, had set up in 1910 the Castle Publishing Co. The premises were behind the 'Post' offices, then in Fishergate, Preston's main street. The company printed Christmas cards for private trade, which extended over the British Empire. Ex-patriots wrote out their messages to be printed, chose the design from a catalogue and the agent liaised with Preston.

Now he told this newly arrived mother that she faced insurmountable obstacles if she chose to bring up her children alone in Australia. He advised her to return to Britain.

No passenger ships were available as all were needed for troops. At one shipping line, when Mrs. Hodkinson sadly turned to leave the office after an unsuccessful attempt to see the Manager, she realised that Mary was missing.

The alarm was raised and a search led to the inner sanctum of the Manager's room where Mary was sitting on his knee telling him all about the naughty man who would not let them go home. Charmed and now helpful, he suggested that they should hurry to re-join the Ionic which was to call first at New Zealand. Cases were re-packed and aboard. The crossing to Wellington was a nightmare of seething seas. Routine medical examination occurred before landing ashore, and on arrival Mary and

Harold were whisked away without their mother's knowledge. It was 24 fraught hours before they were located in hospital. Harold had diphtheria and Mary was diagnosed as a carrier.

The Ionic sailed on. Fortunately their mother could be accommodated during the six weeks of their hospitalisation at the Wellington home of her youngest brother George.

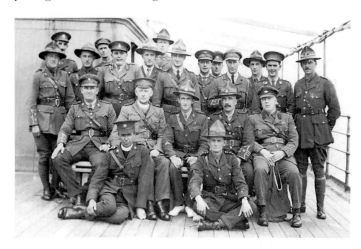

The Officers 39th Reinforcements NZEF Relief Ship Goentoer - August 1918

The Athenic of the White Star Line happened to be taking the 39th reinforcements of the New Zealand Army to Britain and her Captain accepted the now discharged children and their mother together with 1000 men.

The ship was given a rousing send off by a contingent of Maoris clad in tribal finery executing fearsome war dances. They presented Baby Margaret with a statue of a Maori God, a precious souvenir.

After crossing the Pacific Ocean, the Athenic was cheered by crowds lining the recently opened Panama Canal and beautiful Panamanian women in native dress waved the troops on their way.

After some days sailing, as darkness fell the Captain had been instructed to sail between three lighthouses but, unknown to him only two were lit. When the ship sailed along the indicated route it struck a coral reef at Plum Point. Hawsers were fastened and three times it was hauled off, but drifted straight back on to the rocks without a crash. It had been holed and there was a real fear that the vessel would split in two.

The Captain's first consideration was for the safety of the troops so desperately needed on the Western Front, Mrs. Hodkinson was merely advised to keep the family on deck in case the ship broke up.

A shuttle of lifeboats was organised. Due to the tipping of a smaller boat when being lowered from the deck, a soldier fell into the water. He was seized by a shark and never seen again. Attracted by the smell of blood more sharks circled the ship, a sight to unnerve the children. Their mother secured them in their cabin and returned to deck just in time to witness a second soldier fall. A shark almost caught him but he was pulled to safety by one of his comrades.

Mrs. Hodkinson, realising with horror that they had no lifebelts, she could not decide whether to leave the children whilst she searched for belts, or should she take them with her? If the ship split in half she might never see them again. She sank on her bunk trying to make an impossible decision. Then a wonderful thing happened. Trained to iron self-control and rational action this courageous follower of Swedenborgian precepts was granted a vision. She saw Joseph, her late husband, walk across the water, sit down beside her and assure her everything would be all right. It amused her children when grown that the army chaplain no favourite of their mother, had come along and said the same thing.

After five days on the reef, the exhausted mother who had spent hours trying to settle the children to sleep would now have to wake them in the night: the Captain sent information that the family and crew were to be disembarked leaving only a skeleton crew aboard. The news acted like a release valve and all a mother's repressed emotions emptied in a gigantic fury. The usually calm, collected and dignified parent rushed around in a rage grabbing cups, plates, teaspoons - anything as booty to compensate for the terrors of the five dreadful days. More than 77 years later all three children survived owning as a memento of the Athenic a single spoon, all that was left of the unlikely hoard, bearing the logo of the White Star Line.

The sail by lifeboat to Kingston went without incident, although 4 year old Harold lost his cap and had severe sun-stroke. At the foot of the Blue Mountains, orchids, hibiscus and bougainvillea bloomed. Lieutenant Nickeas, a Preston man, (his descendants still live in the suburb of Penwortham in the 1990's), was Liaison Officer to the 39th Reinforcements, offered the family the use of his quarters at the Naval Base, while he moved in with his men.

Later the British Consul paid all the expenses of the move to the Montague Hotel in the cooler climate of the foothills. The building with a mirrored dining room was set in a beautiful terraced garden. Floors of natural wood shone brilliantly, polished by male and female Jamaicans using banana skins. Bringing their own food with them they started work at 5 a.m. and earned five shillings (25p) weekly. The children loved the happy Jamaican people, especially their Ayah who cared for them whilst their mother went sightseeing and shopping. Mary remembered an expedition which she shared, to buy voile, which was made into white shift dresses for the little girls, adorned with embroidered medallions, one on the bodice and one on the skirt.

This Jamaican idyll lasted until the relief ship Goentoer, a Dutch ship of the Rotterdamsche Lloyd Line, enveloped them. For safety on such a large vessel if a naval incident had arisen, each child was allocated a military escort. Margaret not yet two, had a Private, Harold was put in charge of a Corporal and Mary now nearly six years old enjoyed the attentions of an Officer and set her sights high ever after.

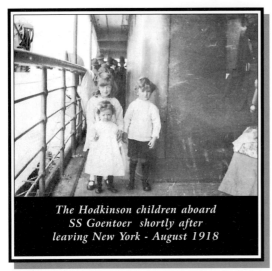

The Hodkinson children aboard SS Goentoer shortly after leaving New York - August 1918

At New York the vessel was to join a convoy that would protect them during the hazardous trip across the Atlantic. They arrived there at night but Mary was allowed to go up on deck as they drifted past the Statue of Liberty, its blazing crown out-shining the stars in brilliance. Whilst awaiting the convoy the family, as civilians, were allowed ashore, to wander in Times Square past huge notices proclaiming that the United States was winning the war. People were singing 'Over There' the U.S. popular song of both World wars.

The Goentoer was ordered to rendezvous at Newfoundland with the convoy. U-boat patrols compelled them to seek safety in New York harbour several times before the convoy could maintain a protective presence on the horizon, and the Goentoer zig-zagged across the Atlantic darting back and forth to deflect enemy torpedoes. Occasionally a destroyer sailed alongside as low in the water as a minesweeper while the bulky Goentoer towered above like a Colossus. After nearly nine weeks they sailed into Liverpool on 3rd September 1918.

Protected by Providence and supported by their wonderful mother, this strange sea voyage set the children up for life, and even the once sickly Harold bloomed.

Ionic   built 1902 Harland & Wolf, Belfast.
                 7812 nett registered tons
                 Service from U.K. to N.Z. 1932 Tourist class only
                 1937 Left Liverpool for Osaka (Japan) to be broken up

Athenic   built 1902 Harland & Wolf. 7826 nett registered tons
                 121 1st class; 117 2nd class; 450 3rd class
                 1928 Sold to Norwegians to be whaling mother ship
                 1941 captured by German cruiser in the Antarctic; used as experimental vessel by 24th U-boat Flotilla in Norway
                 1944 sunk at Kirkenes
                 1945 Raised by Norwegians and served again as whaling ship
                 1962 broken up at Hamburg

Goentoer   Rotterdamsche Lloyd Line

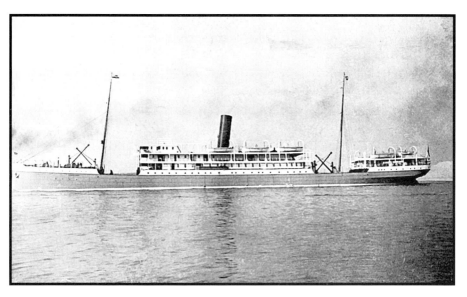

SS Goentoer relief ship H.M.T. Authenic - August 1918

Growing up in Preston

The air in the outer estuary of the tidal River Ribble at Preston might share some of the purity of the water in the open sea, but in 1918 the town on its northern bank that now welcomed the family had within its boundaries 40 coal-powered weaving mills and 6 cupola foundries. Curtains, window-sills, back yards and front flags were regularly washed by women who were also often working long hours in the mills.

Mary's elderly grandparents lived at No. 11 Wren Street in Deepdale in the north east of Preston. The neat complex of streets with bird-names was locally known as Canary Island. The area had been adopted by the Borough in 1914 so the roads had stone sets and the pavements were flagged. This late nineteeth century development by private builders reflected in its more generous proportions the alarm felt by the authorities concerning the high mortality rate in the town

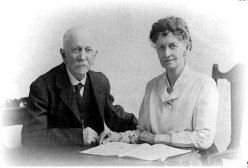

Mr & Mrs Thomas Clarkson.
Mary's Grandparents c.1921

which could no longer be ignored beyond the 1870s. These three-up, two-down terraced houses, had a single storey extension for the scullery, W.C. and washhouse.

The luggage was to follow, when unloaded from the Goentoer, so after the train and tram journey from Liverpool, Mrs. Hodkinson approached the end house in Wren Street by the high back yard door which was in Goldfinch Street. She quietly lined the children up behind her, and knocked on the scullery door. The grandparents did not even know the family was safely back in England so in the neat kitchen, with its black cooking range surmounted by its chenille bobbled mantelcloth there was great rejoicing and thankfulness.

It was September 1918, a few days before Mary's 6th birthday. The space and comparative affluence of her first home in Wigan, the vast expanses of sea, land and sky on the 'Grand Tour' had given her a beckoning vision of possibilities symbolised by 'Daddy's Star'. The world was full of change, opportunity and enjoyment.

The children were blessed in their Grandmother Clarkson who, after bringing up her own six children, was now welcoming a family of four into her small house. She was willing to supervise the children when their mother was out at work but her daughter must retain moral responsibility.

Mrs. Clarkson's family had come from Colne, East Lancashire. In 1865 she, Nancy, was assisting her Aunt Brown in Blackpool managing Brown's Hotel. Her own mother had married into the Ayre family, one branch of which ran a printing business, another were builders. Streets of houses they built in Blackpool bear the names of Mary's great-uncles. Miss Nancy Ayre (known at the time, with a certain status, as Miss Ayre of Blackpool), married in 1877 Thomas Clarkson a drysalter from Kirkham. After a move to Ulverston, where Mary's mother was born, they returned to the Fylde and Preston. Mary's now retired grandfather was a happy-go-lucky playfellow, as Mary remembered, counterbalancing the sterner authority of his wife.

200 yards from the yard door in Goldfinch Street, Deepdale School had been opened in May 1910. Two terms later Miss Charlotte Struthers as head of the Infant School presented to the Manager," a magnificent report." In 1927 when she left a high standard had been set.

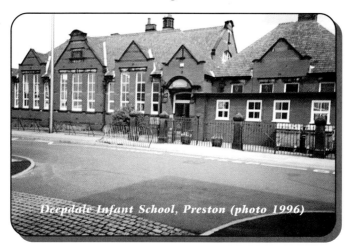

Deepdale Infant School, Preston (photo 1996)

All the teachers were women except the Head of the Mixed Department, Mr. S. Parkinson. Frugality ruled and maleness being rewarded by a higher salary until after the Second World War, gifted women teachers were a good bargain.

Miss Struthers embellished the classrooms with framed pictures "On loan from the Harris Free Public Library and Museum." In her log book she recorded the shining physical cleanliness at the start of the school year. The first caretaker had been selected from 338 applicants. Henceforth the School's birthday was celebrated with pride and pomp, "all the lessons centred round it."

Her book "Number plays and games for infants" (Stepping stones in visual and observational arithmetic series, published by Pitman in 1912) is illustrated by photographs of arithmetic in action in Deepdale School yard.

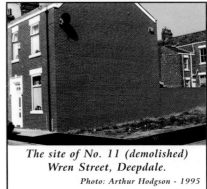

The site of No. 11 (demolished) Wren Street, Deepdale.
Photo: Arthur Hodgson - 1995

In 1912 there is a note in the log about "Control of Staff" with a list of "Duties." She adds " We are not yet ready for "Freedom." This control was the brace behind enlightened methods, such as the experiment "how the children can teach each other." The log entry for the 31st July 1912 includes "work in all classes will be of an informal character, especially the Reading, Writing and Number lessons."

Late in 1918 five changes of staff occurred, as Forces personnel were beginning to return from the Battle Fronts. The two elder Hodkinson children were admitted to the same class shortly before the November Armistice. Neither child had had any professional schooling before. Before the teacher had noticed Harold rolling a cotton reel over the top of his desk, Mary explained his inattention "It's all right. He will be better in a few days. He has been very poorly." Harold's weak health was now only a useful excuse while coughs, colds, sore throats ravaged other local children not invigorated by a world tour. On 1st April 1919 the weather was "intensely cold, ground covered with snow." At last on 17th May the sun: lessons were conducted out of doors and on the 14th July, Saturday, the teachers took their classes to the Great Peace celebrations on nearby Moor Park.

In 1920 and 1921 Miss Struthers introduced Montessori methods but not "wholly" as the "teachers have difficulty in interpreting the principles - but by degrees the power will come."

Hers was the only infants department to display in the 1922 Preston Guild. The children were dressed representing nursery rhymes. Mary's shy little sister took part, and remembering Miss Struthers ample frame reports "she was cuddly too." The great Avenham Park pageant drew a remark from an American visitor reported in A. J. Berry's *Historical Pageant. Preston Guild 1922.* "It beats all our parades over yonder."

There was intelligent control at Mary's home too. Her grandfather said "If you can read that page by the end of the week I will give you a penny". Did Harold have to achieve this too? Yes, but he would get sixpence, when word perfect. Mary received her penny; she asked why she received only a penny and her brother was offered sixpence. Answer: "I knew I would have to pay you." A very important lesson was learned.

The heavy household chores which the children shared gave many opportunities for Grandmother's moral lessons. Mary's most regular duty twice daily was standing on a little stool at the slop-stone in the scullery doing the washing up in a large iron pot. Grandmother carried hot water from the boiler at one side of the coal fire in the kitchen-living room. Mary's work had to be perfect, dishes dried, sink washed and the iron pot set on the draining board. One day a greasy ring was found at the bottom of it: Mary was horrified at her own negligence.

One day the meal having taken longer than usual, she asked to go, to be in time for school. A blank refusal - "Finish one job at a time and be punctual." Cleanliness and punctuality : lessons of inestimable value in a nursing career.

When Mary, as a bright and interested pupil, had been moved to a higher class it was her turn to administer justice. The quick temper, one of her characteristics at that time, was justly used when a boy was treated unfairly after being behind with his work after hospitalisation. The victimisation by the teacher, commenting on his stupidity and mannerisms, had escalated until Mary could endure it no longer. She stood up in class and told the woman teacher to leave him alone, adding the medical rider "how would you like to have seven foot of your bowel removed?" Later Mary's mother learned that the teacher's father, a civic dignitary, spent much time with his cronies, often returning home drunk in the early hours of the morning. He was known on occasion to turn out from the house in their nightclothes, his helpless wife and daughter. This made more understandable the teacher's hardness to the boys in her class. When Mary held a position of authority she insisted on investigating a human problem on all sides.

Mary had strong motivation to win a Borough Council Scholarship to be able to attend the Park School, a grammar school for girls in Moor Park. Seeing a Park School girl cycling on a windy day, wearing a panama hat (with the Preston coat of arms) which billowed behind on its elastic like a halo, had been an inspiring vision.

When she was seven years old, being questioned as to what she would like to be, her immediate response was "To be the first woman Prime Minister of England." Her mother was a member of the Liberal Party but encounters with family who were of the Labour persuasion, taught Mary how to discuss without rancour, to be sure of facts and to accept correction or another's point of view. The empowerment of women was of political interest at this time. To converse sensibly and to join in with adults was encouraged at all times.

The auspices for a bright child in a fatherless family were not good. The Depression was evident. Miss Struthers reports "The whole of this week I have taken standard 1B with Miss A Breakall (student) to demonstrate methods with slow delicate children" (3rd Feb. 1922). "Standards 1A & B tested, 13 children all over eight years old cannot read at all, 3 Deepdale children and 10 new children from Holme Slack. These appear to have had no settled homes and so got very much neglected."

On that same day (4th June 1923) the Head of the Mixed School, Mr. Ward, recorded that 6 selected scholarship girls went for oral test at the Park School. The eager child from Wren Street spoke out clearly - so before her 11th birthday, Mary was awarded a grammar school place. The Borough's policy, advanced by Preston's Director of Education Mr. A. J. Berry, made provision for books and uniform, the cost of which could be insurmountable even for an ordinary family.

Mary owed much of her balanced view of life to the magnanimity and consistency of her early mentors. Her confidence in her own power was never shaken. At the Park School, in an informal class magazine a witty young contributor had characterised its members. Mary's adolescent personality gained the entry "Make me greater, make me greater, ten times greater than the others." This was the Struthers philosophy with extras: "by degrees the power will come."

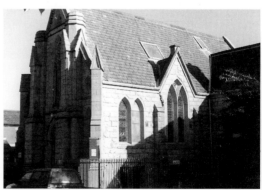

*The New Church
(Swedenborgian),
Avenham Road, Preston.*

Photo: Arthur Hodgson - 1995

One Parent Family

The power behind her children's achievements was Mrs. Hodkinson. On arrival in Preston in 1918 she had obtained immediate employment at Billington's in Glovers Court, a firm specialising in engraving. Not only did silver cups and trophies receive ornate inscriptions; business plates, wedding and engagement rings and silver cutlery were engraved. She left the house at 8.0. a.m. but however late home in the evening she always gave her attention to her children before they went to sleep.

When Mr. Billington gave up the engraving business of which he was manager, Mrs. Hodkinson needed other employment. The only work she was offered at the Labour Exchange was in a fish and chip shop from 6.0 p.m. to 11.0 p.m., quite unacceptable to a mother who desired as much contact with her children as possible.

So it came about that her brother Jack's involvement in the Castle Publishing Christmas card business consolidated the children's knowledge of an ancient part of Preston with family connections. The business had been established in 1910 by George Toulmin who later became Sir George Toulmin. Access to Castle Yard where the premises adjoined the *Lancashire Daily Post* office was by Anchor Court an alleyway off the Friargate end of Cheapside in Preston's town centre. On the corner was a hotel, The White Horse, where the Hodkinson children loved to collect beef dripping to spread on their bread. It was where their Mother's youngest brother George had trained as a chef before emigrating to New Zealand. He had assisted the family there in their 1918 trek around the World.

Mrs. Hodkinson was employed in the office at Castle Publishing Co. which also required help with the seasonal pressures and in the spring preparing the sample books of private Christmas greeting cards to be sent to agents both at home and abroad; then preparing the orders sent in by agents for the printers and the packing department. There were long hours at the office during the weeks leading up to the Christmas season.

Much of the work was craft work that her children could understand and occasionally 'help' with. Mary remembered inserting the coloured ribbons in the cards.

When Harold was 14 he was apprenticed to the printing trade and became expert in the use of the die-stamping machine, a raised printing process used for printing business cards and letter headings for professional people, lawyers, doctors and accountants.

To ensure that there was no lack of exclusive, unleaked marketable designs and verses for the next Castle sample book, social intercourse between the lively Hodkinson children and their cousins in Accrington, whose parents were in the same trade, was discouraged between the months of January and March. A unique 'perk' of the job was the spare end-of-roll newsprint paper which their mother bought for sixpence from the adjacent newspaper office, its tall white presence in a corner at home offering generous use of it.

The job with Uncle Jack gave security but no affluence. Mrs. Hodkinson's house-keeping and dressmaking skills, manifest when she invited him to tea to press for more than the original 30 shillings a week, gave him reason never to increase her wage. Only several years later was it increased to £2 per week.

A few days before Christmas the children had walked, as they often did from Wren Street in Deepdale, to meet their mother. Whilst she was delayed for another hour, Uncle Jack produced his Christmas 10 shilling note (50p). He gave it to Mary who led the younger two off to Woolworth's to buy some presents. When they showed their mother, her face dropped as she had come to rely on this regular donation to provide Christmas food. But she showed her approval that the children had bought for others.

The sixpenny box of dominoes for Uncle Harold's family gave pleasure for years afterwards. Mother put no damper on the walk home through the gas-lit streets, across the covered market, Lancaster Road, North Road to Meadow Street, lined with small shops selling all manner of goods, clothes, food, fruit and vegetables, sweets, chemists, with tall coloured bottles in the windows, all with attractive window displays especially at Christmas time. Then on to Deepdale Road, past the Royal Infirmary and home to Grandmother and Grandfather.

Saturday afternoons she devoted to them entirely, usually with walks into the surrounding countryside. A single line train ran to Longridge 5 miles away to the hills, with stops at Deepdale (near home), Goosnargh, and Grimsargh villages. This gave much variety. The child who made a fruit drop last the longest sucking slowly and gently was awarded an extra one.

The New Jerusalem Church in Avenham, west of the town, to which the family walked a mile back and forth at least twice on Sundays was geared to the education of children. After an assembly in the main hall which was in the basement, notices were given out and the register called, the Sunday School classes divided according to age. After the age of 13, classes were of the discussion type. Parties and dances filled winter days, and summer visits to farms were arranged. The Sunday morning service in the Church was rather like an Anglican service, with prayers, hymns and sermon. The children were not 'put out' during the sermon: mother's fruit drops then came in to action.

There was a piano in the parlour at Wren Street. Emily Nelson, a Preston schoolteacher and her mother's cousin offered to give piano lessons to Mary at no charge. So Mary continued her musical education begun in the large upstairs drawing room at Wigan where her father had been building the organ.

Grandpa Clarkson loved music-hall and when work was done there was no restriction on songs around the piano or in the use of the later acquired 'cat's whisker' wireless on which one could receive programmes chiefly from the Manchester region. Reception from America caused great excitement. These refinements came very late in the 1920's.

For a short time Wren Street housed an upright royal piano. An exchange for grandmother's piano had been ordered through a Mr. Danson, whose son had a local radio shop. The order was misunderstood and a grand piano was delivered to the shop. Mr. Danson meanwhile loaned to Wren Street an upright model from stock. Inside the lid was a plate 'Made for Kaiser Wilhelm 11' for use in one of his castles. The correct order came - again a German piano which, after the break-up of her Mother's home Mary kept in store at Blackpool until the charges defeated her small wartime budget.

When Mary was almost eight, Grandfather, after a road accident, developed carcinoma of the tongue due to the impact on a decayed tooth. She helped feed him when he was nursed at home, but he survived only a few months, dying in June 1921 aged 71.

The funeral cortege lined up outside No 11 Wren Street. Family and neighbours had paid their last respects before the lid was screwed down on the coffin where he lay, seeming to Mary to be fully dressed in a dark suit. His sisters and cousins, older grandchildren in addition to friends and neighbours made a large group of mourners. The ladies of the family wore white with hats and dresses trimmed with black and black shoes and handbags. Mary thought it was a beautiful orderly sight as they moved off to the New Jerusalem Church in Avenham.

Later, Mary aged about 10 had another responsibility: to accompany her 75 year old great aunt to be 'minded' at Rushden, near Kettering. She managed the changes of train at Crewe and Northampton with the aplomb of a world traveller. To escape from the bed she shared with the old lady needed more skill: by sucking striped humbugs with a particularly powerful obnoxious smell, she was allowed to leave the bed early. She won the right to help in her cousin's chemist's shop where they were guests, a special treat being the dispensing of five little Beecham's pills from a large container into tiny boxes.

Twelve months after Mr. Clarkson died, Grandmother's mental confusion set practical problems. There was much housework to do and the fireguard had to be locked in place for safety before Mary could set off for school. The deterioration was gradual but that burden was increasingly Mary's. Even the Uncles could not cope and sent Grandmother back home, after a stay with one of them. The doctor was concerned for II year old Mary's health.

In January 1925 Mrs. Hodkinson had managed to raise, by cash surrender of an endowment policy, the deposit to the Borough for a mortgage on a three bedroomed house, No. 40 Symonds Road. It had a back garden and Mrs. Hodkinson delighted in the three beech trees each side of it. When they left New Zealand the precious parting gift which had been given to the infant Margaret, now had its place. It was a wooden emblem for good luck 'Kiaora', screwed on the newel post in the small hall of the new house.

On the day of the move from Wren Street Mary, not yet 13, and the younger Harold had been left behind to scrub every floor in the house, including the outdoor lavatory floor, and the pot in the sink. This was the usual procedure when a respectable family vacated a rented house.

Grandmother's health deteriorated. The matron at Sharoe Green Hospital, still known then as the 'workhouse', had a daughter at the Park School, in the same form as Mary. Matron knew the family had done everything possible and accepted Grandma as patient. If any payment was made it would be by the Friendly Society of Oddfellows, Mary's mother being a member. The standard treatment for such a patient was containment in a cot bed and sedation by morphine. Mary was allowed to visit her and made her usual quick observation of her surroundings.

On the 1st September 1927 both Mary and her mother were preparing to attend a ball. It was Mary's first and she was ready early. Her mother had made her dress with a pocket handkerchief skirt of white and pink panels ending in points at the hem.

Mrs. Hodkinson was upstairs donning her own 'new-length' pink georgette dress when the expected taxi came. But this was an unexpected taxi sent by the hospital to take her to her mother's bedside. Mrs. Clarkson died next day. She was 76.

The ball at the Public Hall -formerly the Corn Exchange- was to celebrate the completed sale (for £5 million) of the *Lancashire Daily Post* to Provincial Newspapers.

Uncle Jack worked with the Toulmin Bros., owners of the *'Post'*. Before leaving for the hospital himself he warned Mary at the dance not to breathe a word about Sharoe Green. Although it was the Municipal Hospital, the connotation of the 'workhouse' lingered on.

Due to their domestic situation Headmistress Miss Stoneman sympathically advised Mrs. Hodkinson, then in indifferent health, to allow Mary to give up the idea of qualifying for teaching. At less than 16 years of age she had matriculated, gaining enough academic certificates to qualify for entry to any profession. But she must put herself on the labour market forthwith.

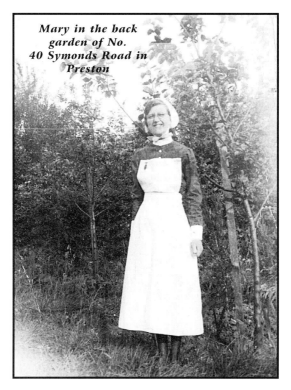

Mary in the back garden of No. 40 Symonds Road in Preston

Teenage Work and Play

In the year after the General Strike it was not easy to find work especially in a town hit by the declining cotton industry. Boots Chemists offered Mary a job on the fancy goods counter. Each counter had its own buyer and three underlings. A small wage was expected to be augmented by commission on certain items, according to a scale of sales difficulty. Furthermore, there was a staff seniority system: when a customer approached, the buyer moved forward first and had the opportunity of the major share of commission. As Mary was the fourth in line she did not move forward very often and her commission was negligible.

She leapt at the opportunity of work at the cash desk. When a return to the fancy goods counter was in the offing she decided to move on elsewhere. She was nineteen.

She found temporary work as a clerk with the Ministry of Labour in the recently built new premises in Pole Street. When she was unsuccessful in the qualifying examination for the Civil Service, she signed on for the 'dole' which was then ten shillings (50p) a week for a limited period only.

Mary was the first in the queue to be interviewed for a job as clerk to Mr. Evan Woodhouse, a motor dealer. He interviewed no more applicants and offered her twenty seven shillings and sixpence per week.

Mary's mother had told her to suspect any job which paid more than £1, and when she discovered that she was to be in an office adjoining a workshop full of mechanics with only the dealer to guide her, her fears of sexual harassment were intensified. Mr. Woodhouse shrewdly suggested that he buy an Alsatian dog, a breed fashionable at that time. The puppy was trained to lie across Mary's doorway. She took the dog home at week-ends.

Mr. Woodhouse's profitable business exploited the trade in fleets of buses which had to be depreciated after seven years service, He could buy them for £30 each for a fleet of seven. The mechanics stripped the bus bodies and built haulage bodies on to the chassis, engines were re-bored, tyres re-moulded and paintwork re-sprayed: the vehicle was now offered at £375. Hire purchase was agreed for a monthly sum. If only one payment was missed the vehicle was repossessed and re-sold.

Mr. Woodhouse became ill with TB meningitis, a lethal illness. He bought the Royal Oak public house at Longridge as a business for his wife and daughter and tried to find another post for Mary. When he was in hospital his partner Fisher Renwick (an importer and exporter from Manchester) cancelled the cash payment to Mrs. Woodhouse, which Mary had been instructed to make, and closed down the Woodhouse business.

Mary, mindful of her own widowed mother's difficulties - the last faint letter in her father's signature on a hurriedly drawn up last testament had seemed to expire with his last breath - went into Mr. Woodhouse's office and extracted a crucial letter proving that Fisher Renwick had broken the partnership by his action. He was now, by law, obliged to stamp Mr. Woodhouse's insurance card from the date he opened the business, thus making his widow eligible for a pension.

Recreation.

During her teen-age years Mary had plenty of youthful company at home and at church. The boy members had set up cycling, swimming and rambling groups.

When up to twelve young people came to the Symonds Road house, on Sunday evenings, Mrs. Hodkinson would have prepared three dozen jam tarts and left the group alone, betaking herself to the sitting room with a book. At 9.45 p.m. she would emerge and ensure that every girl visitor had an escort to the front door of her own home. The group had enjoyed what was the equivalent of a jazz session. It was the time of the Big Bands on the wireless. Fred Steele, whose father had a joinery business in North Road, later became a teacher in London. He was a pianist and made his own one-string fiddle. He and his brother Eric became lay preachers in the New Jerusalem Church. Walter Hunniball, another regular at Symonds Road qualified as a chartered accountant and later became General Manager of Ribble Motors. John Molyneaux was another pianist trained in cabinet making and after the war (serving in the Norway campaign) he started a photography business in Blackburn. Harold Moizer, who came along as John's friend, was a good violinist. Symonds Road introduced him to jazz. He taught himself the saxophone and brought vigour to the Regent dance hall in Tithebarn Street. He later became a woodwork teacher at Kirkham Grammar School. Another boy with his father's help made a microphone. Tom and Leslie Shaw whose parents were caretakers at the Church were regulars. Mary's brother Harold played the drums. The wonderfully tolerant Mrs. Hodkinson won the affection of these young church people, two of whom were killed in action during the 1940's.

Summer rambles included the 22 miles May full moon overnight walk through the Trough of Bowland. It started at Chipping, with Saturday evening fish and chips at 10.0 p.m.. There was no made road through the pass in the 1920's and early 30's, one waded through fords. There were gates at the shallow fords manned by respectable tramps expecting a half-penny or a penny. They might be educated men who were evading a settled life and would cook a walker's own bacon and eggs in a shepherd's hut. The boys might go upstream for a morning bathe. The walk finished at Scorton, then on to the A6 road for the bus through Garstang to Preston. Mary's mother had prepared a hot meal for her family and after a bath and a rub down with olive oil they were ready to walk the mile to church.

Harold was apprenticed, and her sister Margaret was doing well at the Harris Institute Commercial College. In the depths of the recession in the textile industry in 1929/30 things could have been far worse for a fatherless family.

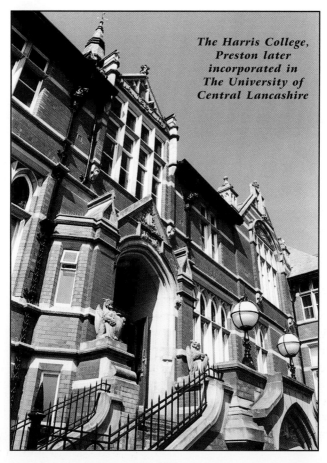

The Harris College, Preston later incorporated in The University of Central Lancashire

Coming of Age 1933
Too Egalitarian for Highgate Hospital
Superb training at North Middlesex Hospital.

Highgate Hospital

After various experiences in local jobs, Mary was now to gain entry to the profession which was to bring her life-long fulfilment.

She scanned Situations Vacant in the newspaper and noted that attendants were needed at the East Wing, Sharoe Green Hospital at Preston. But realising that Mary was worth a full training, a District Nurse friend of Mrs. Hodkinson passed on copies of the *Nursing Mirror*. Training was expected to be done at least 5 miles away from a girl's home area for the sake of patient confidentiality.

In late November 1933 Mary applied for a trainee nurse's post where she would be paid a wage at Highgate Hospital run by the London County Council. For the first three months of appointment a trainee was on probation, known as a 'Whitecoat' and paid £18 per annum with board and lodging.

Since 1929 when the workhouse hospitals had been taken over by the Municipalities, a girl without means, given stamina and endurance, could work her way to full training. Highgate Hospital was one of these.

Things were quite different in the Voluntary Hospitals, such as The Florence Nightingale Training School, where probationers paid a premium for the privilege of training. At Guy's Hospital as 'ladies' they took their personal maids with them to do the more menial work.

Mary began on the 15th December. Working conditions were appalling and there was a high turnover of dissatisfied staff, but at the age of 21, Mary was more mature than many entrants and could cope.

Her working day began at 7. 0 a.m. and ended at 9.0 p.m. with 2 hours off during the day. Whilst sweeping floors, washing up, cleaning lockers and feeding patients, Mary would exchange a few friendly words with the beds' occupants, most of whom, chronically sick, were unlikely to recover; this girl from the North could not accept that therapeutic social intercourse was against the rules. After 3 months she took the written test, and Matron interviewed her saying, "I am afraid I am going to require you to do another month before I decide whether to take you on for training.

With regard to your work, Sister Tutor says you have done excellently in your written paper but that you "TALK TO THE PATIENTS". Mary replied: "I don't stop working". "Yes, Sister says you get through your work very well indeed. But these people are vagabonds and street people - not the sort for you to associate with." Mary replied, "Matron, I understand that nursing levels ALL. Apparently it does not here so I wish to give you my notice."

Once again Mary scanned the Situations Vacant. She must move quickly. The slump in the economy was at its worst. Her situation at Highgate had some advantages: she had board and lodging. It was a safe employment: with employment card surrendered a nurse was exempted from paying any insurance contribution.

Her brother Harold was, like many young journeymen, unemployed and filling in time learning Linotype skills in Leeds, funded partly by the Typographical Association (the Printers' Union). Margaret had completed the two year course at the Harris Institute and was working for 10/- per week for a showcard and poster writer in the town, continuing her studies at evening classes. Mrs. Hodkinson's £2 a week had to stretch far.

North Middlesex Hospital

Another Whitecoat had failed the written test and though she had applied for details of a job at the North Middlesex Hospital she was too young to be eligible so she flung the application form to Mary. Interviews were on Mary's last working day at Highgate Hospital. Fortunately the North Middlesex Hospital accepted Mary's application as a probationer. Pay was £30 per annum. Whenever possible Mary sent £2 a month to her mother.

There, nothing less than perfection was expected in a nurse's performance. Under the Medical Superintendent Mr. Ivor Lewis, surgeon, training was administered not only with military discipline, but like a boarding school of an enlightened type. It was understood that nursing was a vocation and no married woman was employed. The same attitude obtained in teaching in the nation's schools.

Three months were spent in the Preliminary Training School and those who passed the examinations were accepted as contract probationers for the next three years. There were lectures every day and practical demonstrations during the first three months before daily duty on the wards.

At the end of the 3 years as a probationer one sat the Hospital examination which was internally moderated. Mr. Ivor Lewis himself lectured and as he believed he was training women rather than mere professionals, his style was to throw oral questions on general matters at probationers. In the written examination there was a compulsory question searching one's alertness about contemporary events - such as the type of turbo- propelled engine in the recently launched Queen Mary.

Following the Hospital examination the probationer sat the State Registration examination without which qualification she could not be employed in a hospital as Staff Nurse, Sister etc. Annual re-registration was required for a two shillings and sixpenny fee.

Mr. Lewis, surgeon and superintendent, opened all the mail himself and if a complaint about a nurse appeared, he set the hierarchy in motion and it was investigated at once. A nurse could be dismissed if she treated herself with an aspirin tablet from the ward or administered the wrong treatment in a minor degree.

The instrument trays had to be set out to a prescribed order; each enema and saline tray required its individual thermometer. On one occasion Mary, noticing that a nurse's tray contained a broken thermometer, handed hers from her own tray as a replacement. Matron on her rounds noticed this, reprimanded Sister and Mary was required to go to Matron's office the next morning to tell her everything regarding the patient with whom she had been working.

Superintendent Lewis believed it to be of vital importance that his nurses should have the best of everything for a healthy life. Each had a single room, excellent food, unlimited hot water and 3 outfits of uniform, with a new set every year.

Payment (by a packet of cash) was a formal monthly procedure, performed in off-duty time. The Steward wrote to Matron to ask all staff to attend - in at one door, proceeding along on the side of a table and out by another door.

On the 30th November Mary noticed Home Sister standing supervising bowls and boxes, collecting for Christmas gifts for the administrators. Mary heard "That is for Matron's present - 2 shillings from each nurse" and did a quick calculation that the sum would have amounted to £90. She said "I'm sorry, I have to support my family who are unemployed — I cannot pay", and made a mental note that if she were ever in a position to receive, she would never accept such expected contributions from junior staff.

The social facilities were excellent. There was a Social Club to which one paid threepence per week, which gave access to a good swimming pool at Enfield where life-saving was taught. At the Gaumont Cinema at the end of Silver Street the girls bought side-by-side one shilling and threepenny best seats, and had the pleasure of seeing and hearing Sidney Torch on the Wurlitzer organ.

There was an arrangement with West End theatres to let the hospitals know if there were spare seats. Tickets were sent and whatever price they were, one paid half. Notices were pinned on the board that seating at Drury Lane, Wigmore Hall etc., was available and if duty allowed one selected a ticket.

The Home Sister vetted the nurse's dress before she left for the theatre. Long evening dresses were raised by a waist elastic band for travel on the Underground and coats left in the cloakroom at the theatre. For Mary - Little Tich, Georgie Wood, Frank Benson, Donald Wolfit and celebrities at Wigmore Hall all came at the reduced price.

Even Mary's visits to homes of fellow worshippers at the New Jerusalem Church in Finsbury Park stretched her imagination. She was welcomed, as were all newcomers, by four maiden ladies, the Misses Kerby, who were visited occasionally by Princess Marina, soon to become the Duchess of Kent. Mary met her there and the Princess recommended a book - Gerald Durrell's *The Lemon Tree*. The ladies' acquaintance with the Princess was because they had taught some of the children of the Royal Family of Russia, when they lived there as daughters of a British entrepreneur. Kate, the eldest of the ladies, mindful of her status, received Mary alone in the drawing room of the Finsbury Park house; port and biscuits were served. At one point she briskly rose to change chairs with Mary, saying "You will now need to get the other side of your body warm". The area was later heavily bombed and Mary believed that these dear 'Alice-in-Wonderland' ladies and the dignified world they inhabited were together gone.

The Royal occasions of this period could be fully enjoyed by implementing the right strategy. Mary was good at this - she loved celebrations, and as mother had been married on the day of King George V's Coronation she prevailed upon her to come down to London in 1935 to see the street decorations for the King's Silver Jubilee. Then they went to stay a few days with cousins in Bournemouth.

Mary was on night duty when a year later she was allowed to hear that the "King's life is drawing peacefully to its close". Then the 'wireless' was whisked away from the ward. These hours of duty gave her a morning opportunity to witness the dramatic funeral procession, attended by representatives of the world's Royal Families, with the great military bands, drilled to perfection. The crowd stood 15 or 20 deep - but Mary, still the confident little girl who had toured the world, asked a tall man to lift her 6 to 7 stone above the people so she had a fine view. The nurses would have been in serious trouble with Home Sister if they had not been in bed in good time before night duty, so they pushed themselves in file off the Underground where passengers were packed tight.

Memories of the theatres of action in the hospital mingle with these Royal splendours. The Proclamation of the Kingship of Edward VIII, recorded in the *Morning Post* coincided with Mary's out-patients' duty. There were two days of operations: one for circumcisions, one for children's tonsils, the extraction of these latter small items - later given a reprieve - was much in vogue at this time before the antibiotic era. The cotton and rubber sheets used had to be scrubbed of the copious amounts of blood. Mary worked with a young nurse named Ina Buckett, who appreciated with Mary, as they worked in the sluice, Lady Macbeth's energetic speeches and echoes of Donald Wolfit's voice as the girls cheered themselves with Shakespeare's gory passages.

Strict hygiene was observed; Mary believed there were fewer infections then than in modern hospitals. Dressings were prepared by the night nurse and these were placed in a metal churn, an autoclave, for steaming - the inner container receiving steam through holes like a big fish kettle. Porters brought the sealed drum to the ward.

Night nurses, in any quiet moments of duty prepared the gauze and cotton wool dressings for treatments and these were put in drums to be sterilised. Even the gown worn by the dressings nurse would have steam treatment in the autoclave. The procedure for changing a dressing was lengthy with strict rules for scrubbing up, correct method of trolley setting and 'non touch' technique: everything aimed at prevention and containment of infection. There were fewer nurses on the wards, working longer hours than in present day hospitals.

The North Middlesex Hospital was, at this time, the first in the country to implement a 3 shift system and reduce the working hours from 60 to 48 hours per week. Staffing on the wards overlapped by two hours at changes. On George VI's Coronation Day on Wednesday 12th May

1937 if work was finished at 7.0 a.m. one could go to town. Such Ward Sisters who could be spared were allowed to take up position on the pavement with stool and coffee the night before.

Mary and her four companions could go no further than Green Park on the Underground, then walked, aiming for the procession route. Mary noticed that a tall policeman very occasionally allowed some of the crowd under his arm on to the Mall. Near the Victoria Monument she observed that an opening had been left through which the military bands emerged from barracks. Forecasting that this would later be closed, Mary led her colleagues to a point where they could veer round and fill the front row, where they had a marvellous view and saw the Royal appearance on the balcony at Buckingham Palace later. These night shift staff were supposed to be back for bed at 11 a.m. but on that special day they joined the festivities in the Strand and did not appear until 11.0 p.m. Then at midnight until 9.0 a.m. premature babies had to be fed every 2 hours by pipette. Not a job a nurse could doze over though the shawl was wrapped comfortably round both nurse and babe!

At Christmas the staff dining room (where ward sisters usually had restaurant-type service, juniors sitting at long tables) became a ballroom. The name and address of one's male guest was given to Home Sister. Matron and the Medical Superintendent received all guests formally when presented by the nurse-hostess and then they together led off the first dance when the band struck up. For two years running Roy Fox's band was engaged. They then announced "Now is the time for us to withdraw" leaving the Assistant Matrons in charge. Many of the guests were young doctors from neighbouring hospitals.

In 1937 Mary received her State Registration. Matron approached her in June to offer training in midwifery, for which a £50 fee would be waived if one worked an extra six months on the Chronic Sick ward Mary's mother encouraged her to do this: "Yes midwifery" would be marvellous then you could go out to India and marry a Colonel!" When he was widowed a Mr. Green, a tea planter in Assam had approached the one time Miss Clarkson. She refused on account of her children, his offer of a new life. Perhaps , she now thought, this attractive dream could be fulfilled by her daughter.

But Mary's destiny was influenced by her early childhood in her father's Wigan shop. The watch-maker's and jeweller's business included an eye-testing service and she had worn spectacles herself since the age of

8 when her mother observed that she could not read notices in the doctor's waiting room. She felt complete with her glasses and during war conditions slept wearing them in readiness for emergency action.

She noticed that the Royal Eye Hospital at Manchester was offering training in Ophthalmic Nursing, for a Staff Nurse.

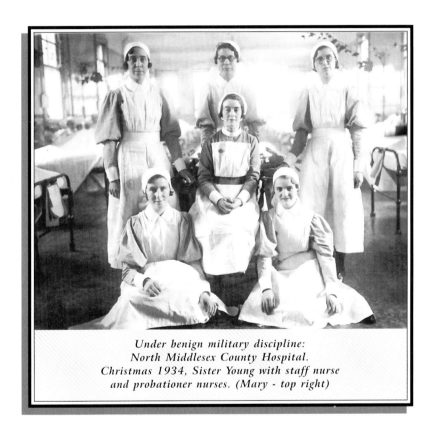

Under benign military discipline:
North Middlesex County Hospital.
Christmas 1934, Sister Young with staff nurse
and probationer nurses. (Mary - top right)

A young professional in Opthalmic Nursing

Royal Eye Hospital, Manchester. 1937-38

Before the end of June Mary was living in the Nurses's Home on Oxford Road, Manchester ready for 60 hours duty per week. Breakfast was at 6.30 a.m., ward duty at 7.0 a.m. One took 2 hours off either morning or afternoon and a half day a week from 2 p.m. Subject to Matron's approval - a nurse had to go and ask - one day per calendar month was conceded. Junior nurses had to be indoors by 8.0 p.m., a Staff Nurse by 9.0 p.m. Night duty was from 9.0 p.m. to 7.0 a.m. Salary was £60 per annum for a Staff Nurse providing her own uniform.

This was the regime of a University Voluntary Hospital, a sister hospital of Manchester Royal Infirmary. It was a teaching hospital and it selected patients who would further the educational aim. The consultants were not paid by the Hospital: remuneration came from private patients. The consultant was granted a group of beds where these patients could be treated experimentally. Doctors, junior doctors and nurses were paying their own fees to be trained There were seven eye hospitals in the country at this period, some of them such as Moorfields boasting a very early foundation.

Lectures to nurses were given by Sister Tutors with doctors giving the occasional one. Sisters sat in for the eye consultants' lectures. The wards were used as a training ground for medical students and junior doctors from the University. The focus was on eyes alone. Mary reported a child with a cough bad enough to be whooping cough but the doctor replied that it was the nurse's job to know about that, not his. Mary could apply her knowledge of the ward routine she had learned at the North Middlesex Hospital.

It was regarding the hierarchy and etiquette that Mary had to be vigilant and re-educated. Junior nurses did not speak to a Staff Nurse unless she spoke first. The situation of a Staff Nurse speaking to other Staff Nurses was more tricky, as their seniority, determined by their date of joining the team of 12, had to be remembered. When one graduated to 11th, one could speak to everyone, as one was allowed to address the one next up as well as those below.

It was easy to distinguish between Miss Duff Grant, Matron of M.R.I. who visited occasionally (she was a Scottish whisky Grant, tall and aristocratic in appearance with an easy familiarity of manner) and Miss Barter, Matron of the Eye Hospital, who was dumpy and wore her clothes as though she had slept in them. Her tiny dog which followed her everywhere (despite hospital rules) was extracted from under the beds by her call "Come to Mother!"

All Matron Grant's nurses were required to wear their hair in a high bun. If their own hair did not provide for this a bun was fitted on, attached to the regulation cap. Matron Barter's nurses sported a bit of feminine frippery with butterfly tails behind the head. Length of dresses must be 2 inches above the ankle.

The Nurse's Home had just been re-built when Mary arrived. It had accommodation for probationer nurses who started their training at 16 years of age, spending two years on ward work. A good educational level was required for entry. Staff nurses brought experience of general nursing and gained speciality experience in the care of eyes. The Sisters were responsible for ward administration and helped with training of all nurses and juniors. The three categories lived in separate sections of the Home. There was a communal sitting room and dining room where nurses sat in position according to the hierarchy. No cigarette could be smoked except in a room furnished with chairs and ash trays on the top floor and one had to change out of uniform before going there.

Oxford Road, Manchester gave easy access to theatre entertainment. When asking for a 'theatre pass', one was lucky to acquire a pass per week and even that, one felt, might be refused. Mary had a taste for music hall and repertory theatre which she, thought, might be suspect areas of interest. 'Sacred' concerts were more highly approved.

The duties of the surgical theatre Staff Nurse were heavy. Most operations were done under local anaesthetics and it was her responsibility to ensure that cocaine in the form of drops was correctly administered. The theatre was heated by a coal fire and it was also her job to see that the right temperature prevailed - without smoke or pollutants. Mary pointed out to Home Sister that theatre Nurse Bowes was suffering from boils, may-be associated with inadequate meals and off-duty time. Matron's office pronouncement to Mary was "I understand you think I am not treating Bowes well! You shall both come with me and have an evening out."

The girls were to make their own way to the 'Sacred Concert', to seats nowhere near Matron. Isobel Baillie was singing and Ian Wallace (Song of the Flea) bass. As they were to return in Matron's taxi they climbed the stairs to see, outside the dress circle, a little woman in hospital uniform, overtopped by a mothy-looking fur coat. She was loudly commanding "I am Matron of the Manchester Royal Eye Hospital "Where is my car?"

But noise in her hospital was a different matter. One day Mary and her colleagues were coming from lunch, laughing and chattering in the corridor. There was a formidable command from behind: "Nurses! I am a Bart's trained nurse. Sister Tutor always told us that a noisy nurse is an abomination, I will not have FOUR ABOMINATIONS IN MY HOSPITAL." The nurses were returning to the ward after eating monotonous fare. The rice pudding served every evening was cooked in big cooking vats, beginning on Sunday as a white mixture. It was warmed up daily until Saturday when it appeared nearly black.

'Voluntary ' status justified extreme frugality, to the extent that nurses off duty in the evening were not allowed supper. When Mary challenged this by sitting down in mufti for the meal the long-serving Assistant Matron was non-plussed; such a thing had never happened before. She cut a square of toast from each of the 11 pieces provided and finished the square off with a baked bean from the twelve beans each apportioned to 11 nurses. There was a slight improvement after this effective protest.

The doctors had a different menu. As a maid was clearing after the doctors' meal the young nurses' eyes were riveted on a small piece of salmon left over. One junior popped it in her mouth. Matron failed to see the funny side and wished to know who had done this: "Who has taken the square inch of salmon?".

At the end of nine months Mary received the highest marks of all Staff Nurses and was awarded the Bronze Medal from the Hospital. She was put in charge of Matron's ward, the ward used by the University. A short corridor led from it to Matron's office, though Matron took no particular responsibility for the ward. Mary's salary was raised to the £90 per year scale.

A dust-free environment was regarded as imperative during the dressing of eyes. On one occasion the Senior Professor Mr. Warton had indicated that he would be making an early round and was annoyed that the patients had not been prepared for him, and reported negligence. Matron had to agree with Mary that hers was the correct procedure: no eye must be uncovered until ward-cleaning was finished.

It was Mary's extra duty to ensure that there was a good supply of Formalin mouthwash for the Professor. He performed operations very successfully with a high quantity of whisky in his bloodstream but in the theatre the aroma was disguised by the Formalin.

Mary's three months on this ward coincided with summer when the Professor's hobby of specialist rose growing led him to bring a gorgeous bunch of perfumed blooms for Matron. Mary overstepped the professional mark by admiring them. Next day when he brought a smaller bunch for her she was summoned to Matron's office to hear "I understand the Professor brought you some roses. They were not for you to admire".

Mary found Matron's unexpected reactions interesting. They were not whimsical but formed by the hierarchical discipline to which she had been subjected herself, trained at 'Barts'.

At Matron's pleasure Mary could have one day off per month. Linked with her weekly half-day this gave her time to go home to Preston. Not realising that the return train was a stopping one she had to knock up an irate Home Sister (in dressing gown and slippers) as she arrived later than the 10.0 p.m late pass allowed. When she went to apologise the following day to Matron (before Home Sister could report her), Matron said "Could you in future be back by 12 noon the following day? " She never granted this concession to anyone else.

Medical treatments too were interesting. Whilst Mary was in charge of the 'University' ward the first corneal graft ever was successfully achieved - not done by one of the most senior doctors but by a Mr. Duthie who performed it with the minimum of suturing.

Publicity, especially personal publicity, was then regarded as beneath the dignity of a noble profession and when the *Manchester Guardian,* hot as usual in pursuit of 'progress', published an article on Mr. Duthie's achievement, he was very annoyed. Another consultant - Mr. Smith - made another breakthrough by going into the cornea itself using more sutures. Mary was allowed to take out the sutures. A clamp was fixed to help keep the eye open. Most of the instruments were fashioned in silver doll's-house-size forceps and small scissors. Mary loved using the dainty pressure scale which she skilfully positioned on top of the eye-ball to measure accurately the degree of pressure which might lead to the disease glaucoma if untreated.

Men patients often presented with eyes affected by coal dust. There was much jocularity when they were expected, when seated, to rest their head backwards on the nurse's chest for her to be able to gently lift the lashes and apply treatment.

Atropine and Pylocarpin were applied to the patients eyes alternately to widen or contract the pupil. If a nurse was leaving duty with widened pupils it was a give-away that she had broken the rule never to touch her own eyes; even traces on the fingers could affect the eye.

Conjuctivitis (a disease prevalent in areas of malnutrition) was treated by hot bathing in the Outpatients' Department. Patients were seated at a long table from which hollows like little bowls were scooped out of the wood. Each person was give a wooden spoon onto the back of which cut-out pads of cotton wool and lint had been carefully bandaged. A supply of steam was piped to the table and as it condensed in the bowls, the patient brought the dipped spoon to the eye.

Another treatment that required much manual dexterity by the nurse was the application to the eye of steam-heated lint. Speed in rolling the lint, using both hands in the process, was essential. Inexperienced and less dexterous nurses acquired heat blisters on their fingers.

Mary now in July 1938 felt experienced enough for a position as Sister.

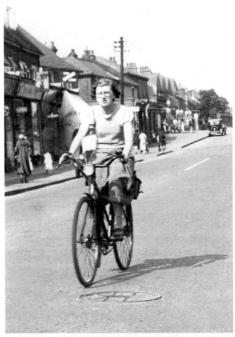

Mary off duty in 1935

Sister; nursing underprivileged children of Birmingham. 1938-1940

An advertised vacancy for a Sister at Birmingham Eye Hospital attracted Mary's attention and an interview was arranged to coincide with a meeting of the Hospital Board. A room crowded with its all-male members opened from Matron's office like an inner trap-box as in a Hans Andersen story. Mary was hustled to a chair behind the door facing the chairman seated at the far end. Before this she had taken a cup of tea alone, no other interviewees in sight.

She learned that the vacancy was not in Birmingham but at Blackwell, in Burcot Grange, a former country house near Bromsgrove, Worcestershire. It was the County Annexe providing a healthy environment in which to recuperate, for the underprivileged of Birmingham.

It was required that patients, many of whom were children, should stay at least a month. For malnutrition and poor living conditions there was no quick treatment. One area of Birmingham, subsequently smashed in the "Blitz", had cottages built round a courtyard, in the centre of which was a furnace used in chain-making and nail-making. A new-born baby might be hung in a hammock near the furnace fire and given a crust of bread soaked in beer to suck.

Matron Saunders supervised all the eye conditions sent from the main hospital; she needed an assistant. General physical conditions were supervised by a local doctor.

Burcot, an isolated place, was approached by the steepest rail incline in the country, and only Big Bertha's engine was strong enough to cope with its heaviest demands. There was no bus service; one walked for basic items the two miles to Bromsgrove.

When the post was offered Mary she replied that without qualified medical attention on the spot, those in charge bore a grave responsibility and she did not consider herself experienced enough for such an appointment. All the Florence Nightingale military administration machine was behind Matron's pronouncement: "If the Committee consider you are competent for this post you ARE." Mary, now just 26 stayed from June 1938 until May 1940.

Ensnared she may have been but the place was beautiful both inside and out. The house had been built as a family home for the affluent Chamberlain family. A double staircase with fine woodwork led from the main hall, lighted on the landing by a large stained glass window depicting happy love scenes from the plays of Shakespeare: nine young couples with the sun behind them.

The Hospital Savings Association also had a home in the grounds. Like many isolated institutions Burcot had its own spirit and atmosphere and the countryside and beautiful leafy lanes of Worcestershire provided constant refreshment.

Matron at Burcot had a cocker spaniel, Judy, and one of Mary's unofficial duties was to take her for a 5 mile daily walk. Judy always knew when it was Mary's day off however much it varied and she would never leave her room door until Mary emerged. It may have been at one time the housekeeper's room. Mary might have her breakfast in the quarters she shared with Matron and always had her evening meal there in the sitting room. It had lovely views as had also her bedroom. The rooms were at the top of the back stairs that led down from the former family bedrooms.

Domestic staffing under the cook/housekeeper was dependent on Welsh girls even as young as 14 or 15. Mary, like Matron, had her own personal maid and became used to "Shall I run your bath?" and having her bed made whilst she was at breakfast.

Pupil nurses from the main hospital would live in for a short time to gain experience working with the staff nurses. The nursing care was friendly, and the therapeutic atmosphere was assisted by the former coachman's accommodation above the coachhouse having been converted to a 3-bedroom flat which could be booked, at no charge, by Sisters on an off-duty week-end from Birmingham Eye Hospital. They could use the dining facilities and professional contact with the Hospital was fostered. The only disadvantage was that theatre-goers must walk the 5 miles back from the City.

The two and a half acre garden, managed by one man and a boy, with a lovely view of the Lickey and Malvern hills was itself restorative. The kitchen garden supplied all the seasonable vegetables to the Main Eye Hospital as well as to Burcot. The superb herbaceous borders on each side of the walled drive were planted in such a way that they could be tended from both sides with tall plants in the centre. A nurse could relax, dead-heading this scented area and pick certain blooms identified by the gardener.

It had puzzled Mary why Matron chose to occupy an attic bedroom rather than the one near the mezzanine quarters she herself used. Someone in the kitchen asked her "Were you not told that the last Sister had committed suicide?" This unfortunate Sister had been horrified that her own illness - scarlet fever- was the cause of children in the annexe contracting it and she was found hanging from the beams of her attic room. Mary confirmed this with Matron who had put the incident firmly in the past but insisted that the room should not be offered to the new Sister.

Christmas was celebrated with the usual hospital enthusiasm. A 70ft decorated tree glistened in the entrance hall. The majority of the extra work fell on the domestic staff. The 2 hours per day free from duty for the little Welsh girls was supplemented by a half day per week and a day off per month and as there were no buses, opportunities for a change of scene were limited. Matron's and Mary's maids were supposed to ensure that all their needs were met before taking a free day.

So Mary devised a special Christmas present for them. The night nurse usually called them in the morning. On Christmas day Mary rose at five, dressed in her uniform, made up a tray in the kitchen and delighted the six girls in their dormitory with tea served at their bedside, so gaining a little luxury to start the special day.

There were happy social occasions when Mary played the piano. On one occasion there was a visitor from Birmingham. A Sister observed this young woman watching Mary and said, "She is in love with you Mary." Mary dismissed this as a joke, as the variety of human behaviour had yet to be learned. The woman asked Mary to accompany her to the theatre in Birmingham and stay the night for convenience in her flat, which Mary did, as she enjoyed good plays. Afterwards in the double bed provided (when Mary strongly repelled her advances) she was asked "Then why did you come?"

On the 3rd September 1939 Matron Saunders and Mary heard the radio announcement and Neville Chamberlain's voice: "This country is now at war with Germany."

Shortly after this broadcast the Secretary of the main Birmingham Eye Hospital telephoned to say that there was to be immediate evacuation from there to Burcot. There were three rings of anti-aircraft guns around the city and Burcot Grange lay between the second and third rings. Soon the stampede of ambulances and cars arrived and mattresses were lined along the floor at Burcot. When after 3 or 4 days the German bombers had still not come, the exercise was performed in reverse.

Meanwhile stocks were being piled by government agencies in the surrounding countryside. Garrisons were filling. The visiting sisters, accustomed to city lights, were intimidated by the black-out but Mary was used to walking in the country lanes in the darkness. After a theatre visit she caught the last train to Barnt Green and walked from there to Blackwell, a distance of five miles, to arrive at Burcot Grange annexe at 11.30 p.m.

Mary's mother had early instructed her girls to carry a rolled newspaper and to walk in the dark in military style. Now soldiers were about in the lanes and when the footsteps approaching in the opposite direction drew near, Mary was amused to hear a male voice exclaim "Blimey it's a woman!"

Having volunteered for the Civil Nursing Reserve Mobile Unit, Mary awaited a call to duty. She decided to take her week-end's leave away from Burcot and being a bit short of cash she arranged to travel on a 'payment on arrival' ticket - to be met by her mother and brother at Preston.

The phoney war dragged on; life seemed in suspense. A young soldier sat opposite to her in the train dragging from Birmingham to Crewe where both changed trains. Their companionship gave him enough confidence to take Mary in his arms on the station platform and kiss her and ask her to write to him. He was Sapper Jack Southward R.E.

They wrote regularly and then Mary heard no more even after the Dunkirk evacuation. Later she had a letter saying that he was in camp at Exeter having been evacuated from Bologne. Mary asked for time off to visit and after a slow journey without any food, except a belated station trolley pie, which made her sick, she managed to contact the camp. Jack had arranged accommodation for her at a nice house in a nearby village and came to meet her. The weather was kind, it was strawberries and cream time and Mary wrote to tell her mother that an engagement to be married was being considered. There was a meeting at Doncaster and several more before a note from Jack stated that his next address would be a British Forces one and gave her his number.

By that time Mary herself had been directed further north in the Civil Nursing Reserve to Lancashire. The Allied Armies were re-forming. When she applied to the War Office for information, they could only pass on a letter from her to Jack as she was not an official correspondent - i.e. a relative. In 1941 she received a note from the War Office to say that Sapper J. Southward was missing believed killed. Mary said reflectively "I would have married Jack Southward."

This was still summer 1940. Matron Saunders at Burcot Grange realised that her deafness would preclude her from Service work and advised Mary to take the post at Bromsgrove where emergency accommodation was established to receive possible military casualties. During the phoney war American volunteers came over and an American unit known as the

American Hospital, Britain No. 1. took over entirely from the British Military at this unit.

In the Bromsgrove unit there were four tables for emergency operations and huge sterilising ovens powered by gas rings. The U.S. doctors' remarks about the provision and equipment was dismissive and patronising. Mary, used to British hospital courtesy, escorting her senior Medical Officer to the door and addressing him as "Sir", scorned the familiarity and tone that the name "Sister" could be made to bear in a loaded accent.

Letters arrived from Margaret who was concerned about her mother's health so Mary took a week-end off to see for herself.

The evening she was due to return to Bromsgrove, her mother reminded her that she had better be moving. Uncharacteristically she postponed this (the Americans could manage!) until the next morning. When her train drew in to Snowhill station, Birmingham, she viewed the wreckage of what would have been her last evening's train. It was also the night of the destruction of Coventry centre, the first big raid outside London which preceded those in Manchester and Liverpool.

At the Bromsgrove Unit she found that not a single patient had been sent and she herself had not been missed. It was time to find a place where she was needed. The young bomb-site waifs from Manchester soon to be gathered into a large house between Preston and Blackpool would be next to receive Mary's skilled devotion to duty.

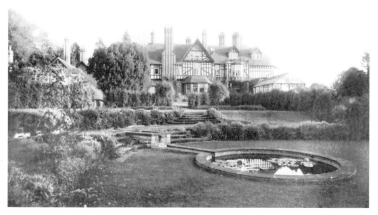

Burcot Grange Annexe of Birmingham and Midland Eye Hospital, opened in 1937. Built by Henry Focett Osler and presented by Mr & Mrs F.W. Rushbrooke. Photo: Birmingham City Libraries.

Ownerless children and a nurse without a memory
The Hill, Westby, Near Kirkham, 1941

In the Civil Nursing Reserve Mary was directed to Kirkham Hospital, near Blackpool (in the 1990's it is Wesham Park Hospital) to find that the military wards were closed due to faulty sanitation. Preferring not to be idle, she approached the Matron of the 'Workhouse' (the name lingering on) as a temporary volunteer helper.

She was appalled by the cursory washing of only hands, face and arms of the bed-fast patients, without even a change of water between each person. With gentle assiduity, necessitating the use of olive oil, she set about cleaning ALL parts.

The Luftwaffe began bombing Manchester just before Christmas in 1940. A month later children, abandoned in air-raid shelters and ruined buildings, were still being found by the emergency services.

A house at Westby, between Preston and Blackpool, named The Hill and under the control of Lancashire County Council, was commandeered as a sick bay for children. Mary, appointed to deal with the arrival of 24 Manchester foundlings aged from 4 to 12 years, had one hour's notice on

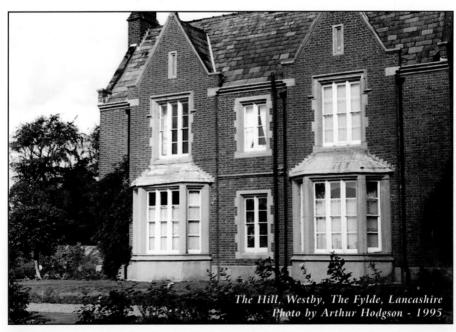

The Hill, Westby, The Fylde, Lancashire
Photo by Arthur Hodgson - 1995

the 21st January 1941. In the kitchen there was a carton of porridge oats, a 2lb bag of sugar, 2 loaves of bread and a cube of butter. A farm supplied milk. A four-plate electric cooker was the only appliance in working order.

These were children for whom the authorities could find no responsible person and who were hazy themselves as to whom they belonged. British children from more careful families during the second world war wore an engraved metal disk attached to outer clothing. The unique number on it denoted one's place of residence and position in the household. Securely owned like a respectably licensed dog, the child remembered its number for a lifetime. Mary had remembered the label fixed to her first world war vest which set such a value on her "alive or dead." At the end of the century during such a discussion about security she would suggest " Ask him if he would like a label."

The Manchester waifs needed nursing care for which the resources were utterly lacking. They suffered from a condition known as 'shelter scabies', erupting like smallpox all over their bodies and needed bathing twice a day. So the hot-plate was constantly in use for heating water. Soiled linen had to be soaked in disinfectant, washed in cold water in the cellar and hand mangled. There was no extra labour. The duration of stay had been intended to be 2 or 5 days. A doctor realised that more help was needed; the Civil Nursing Reserve sent a 36 year old nurse from the Kirkham complex. She was 7 years older than Mary. In Elise May Collin Mary recognised a superb nurse ready for team work. Devising a rota for day and night care was impossible but the two women did it by one beginning at 7 a.m. and working until 3 p.m. when the other had breakfast after some sleep and took over. Both were on call for a four-handed task.

Mary put out desperate appeals for more help. When things were easing off a little, a mature woman, with a lady-of-the-manor style, arrived during a hectic lunch-time, expecting to be received privately in the non-existent Matron's office. She came to offer the occasional assistance not of herself but of another of her own type. No this person could NOT do this, could not do that, but she would be willing to hear the "children's prayers". She departed when Mary answered "If you find me someone to take care of their bodies, the Good Lord will take care of their souls."

The two nurses struggled on alone to the point where Elise collapsed utterly. Mary discovered her in a cupboard suffering from total amnesia. Mary herself was at the point of exhaustion, where she was hallucinating, and she later remembered her vivid waking 'dreams'.

It was Mary's mother who assessed the situation on the spot and went forcefully to County Hall. Within two days the boilers were made to work, a kitchen maid, a cook and full staff were installed. Towards the beginning of March, the two holders of the fort were given their marching orders.

It was then that the partially recovered Elise, re-learning what to do even with a knife and fork by watching Mary, said "You won't let me go into hospital, will you?" Mary replied "As long as I can look after you I will, but I cannot exclude hospital if you need it". It was a promise of care that Mary kept for 46 years. A strange legacy of war; a burden carried cheerfully by a woman not yet 30 years old.

The Hill had been entirely unprepared for resident people so Mary had had furniture including her piano, sent from the Preston home. Now all went into store with Brewer and Turnbull in Blackpool; the two exhausted nurses found accommodation in this town where Air personnel were congregated.

During these hectic days, Mary had gleaned little information about Elise Collin's past, coping with the present took their all. When she came she had handed to Mary for safe-keeping £50 in £5 notes (rarely handled in 1941), two identity cards and a food ration book. When a letter came for Elise, she had asked Mary to accompany her to Blackpool as she had to meet some people there. She asked for the money and identity cards. Mary watched from the Promenade as Elise emerged from the hotel talking to three men. No explanation was offered. She came back to The Hill without the money and with one identity card.

Was Elise's later amnesia assisted by a sworn secrecy? Mary knew she was reluctant to talk about her earlier life. She had come to The Hill from working in the military section of the large mental hospital at Whittingham, near Preston. Much later when Mary was sorting out difficulties with regard to Elise, the bank which Elise had once used in Liverpool informed Mary that she had closed her account at the time of the withdrawal of troops from Dunkirk. This senior man connected her attitude with this - she had been on a hospital ship at an early period of the war which had been torpedoed.

All the evidence Mary had for that from Elise was the quiet remark made by her 40 years later as they watched the TV report of the sinking of the North European ferry The Herald of Free Enterprise - "The worst thing is when the lights go out."

The birth certificate secured when she claimed state pension when she was 60 stated that she was born in 1905 at No. 8 Ferndale Road, Crosby. She was master mariner Horatio Irving Collin's daughter. Was she educated at Malvern High school? There seemed to have been a link.

She had certainly travelled with her father in the merchant service aboard ship calling at East African ports. She had been engaged to be married to a man named 'Reg' who was killed in a motor accident. There was a solitary casual mention of a brother Kenneth connected with a poultry farm in Cheshire. Elise had worked for a doctor in Waterloo, Liverpool. Her mother was Mary Helen Collin, formerly Leatherbarrow.

Elise had the manner and bearing of the old upper middle class; her good educational background and mastery of languages, the mystery surrounding her unwillingness to talk made Mary wonder if she had been used in the Intelligence Services. Her mastery of new skills such as cookery (no domestic training had been given in her girlhood with a nanny and maids) and her easy absorption of a very wide range of facts equipped her to adapt to some expectations of modern practical life. But always the curtain descended, memories were suppressed! Always there was the question Why? to which Elise did not give the answer.

Had she escaped from unwelcome parental expectations, a mother who seemed to be ailing? She had done preliminary nursing training at Saffron Walden Hospital, Essex and passed the examination there. She had held a position at Southwold with a Greek family named Minoprios whose daughter, with learning difficulties, needed nursing care. She was not an S.R.N. but Mary found in her possession a nurse's badge that had a name on it which was not that of Elise. She wrote to the General Nursing Council to locate the owner. The Council forwarded the letter and Mary had a reply from a retired nurse living in Hawkshead, Cumbria. When Mary visited her - her brother driving her there - the lady said yes, she did remember Elise from Whittingham, Preston nursing days, but she said nothing more. Again a veil was drawn.

A few years later and still during the war, Mary noticed discarded wrapping paper on the coal bunker: Elise had had a parcel from 31 Ashlar Road, Crosby. Mary made a note of this and when, much later she had a chance to go there, she found that the occupants of the house had lived there for 13 years and knew of no previous resident named Collin.

The interaction of character, impulse, opportunity and chance are reflected in the emphasis that Mary's spoken recall placed on particular incidents: incidents and memories that have revealed a pattern in the vocation to nurse, to bring health, to give support. The spontaneous selection of memory etched a clear picture. But her assuming responsibility for Elise was passed over without comment. Just as a good soldier would bring a wounded comrade from behind enemy lines, so Mary took on her fellow-nurse disabled by war. "There's a war on" was the catch phrase:

survival and service were all that mattered. There was then no study of battle-fatigue, or post-traumatic stress disorders. There was no field hospital for the treatment of Elise's hidden war-wounds.

By skilful manipulation of opportunities, by realistic expectations and great forbearance, Mary gained many rewards and some respite but she carried the stretcher to the end of Elise's life in 1988. She carried it lightly and with enjoyment. She followed no phantoms nor looked around for more worthy recipients of devotion. At the heart of her character lay this unselfish perception of what is reasonable and possible.

During the nursing of the abandoned children in Lancashire the stronger of the two had pulled the other out of breakdown and had made a promise. To understand the binding of that promise we look to Mary's upbringing. Her mother when widowed, brought up the fatherless children the way the father wished. She had promised and 'his star' supported her.

In a rush of spontaneous affection during adolescence Mary had put her arms round her mother. Instead of a laugh and a hug back her mother said "Mary, if you love me show me!" She meant that dedication of action and thought - helpfulness was the way to do it. Ever after Mary wondered if she was 'showing' enough, the way her mother would like to be shown. Was this Mary's Achilles heel instinctively exploited by a neurotic, selfish older Elise?

Swedenborgian values and training

Though great demands were placed upon the individual there was no element of fear in the Swedenborgian training which influenced Mary on her actions. Emanuel Swedenborg (1688-1772) was the son of a bishop in the Lutheran Church, a pious and learned professor of theology in Upsala. His gifted son was a scientist, an engineer, an anatomist and statesman. He was a biblical scholar who stressed the importance of religious freedom and human rationality. He founded no particular sect but meetings of followers soon after his death led to the start of separate institutions in Britain and overseas based on Swedenborg's writings for the Christian church.

Both father and son laid great emphasis on the cardinal virtues of faith, love and communion with God. As an anatomist, Swedenborg's work is recognised as being well to the fore in regard to both the brain and to the ductless glands.

In middle age he was prompted to psychical and spiritual inquiry. Swedenborg claimed to have learnt by his admission into the spiritual world the true states of men in the next life, the scenery and occupation of heaven and hell, true doctrine of Providence, the origin of evil, the sanctity and perpetuity of marriage and to have been a witness of the "last judgement," or the "second coming of the Lord, which is a contemporary event." "All religion" he wrote "has relation to life and the life of religion is to do good." "The Kingdom of Heaven is a kingdom of uses." *

His writings exercised a great influence over S.T. Coleridge, Robert and Elizabeth Browning, Coventry Patmore, Henry Ward Beecher and Thomas Carlyle; also read by the American transcendentalists such as R. W. Emerson.

The New Jerusalem Churches tended to be established in Britain where there was an emergent intellectual and technological middle class. In Accrington, Lancashire, the Society of the New Jerusalem Church was formed in 1802.

Sunday schools were fundamental to the Church's organisation and they acted on Swedenborg's *True Christian Religion* Chapter 7, section 11: "The recreations of charity are feasts and social intercourse".

Feasts and social intercourse were not the terms used by Mary when as Matron she asked Committees for the requirements to rehabilitate the elderly, but they were foremost in her armoury in the battle against apathy, depression and decline.

To the end we sat with Mary at the feast of life. She 'showed' us. Her mother's great expectations were more than fulfilled.

* *Quotations from Encyclopaedia Britannica 11th edition. Vol.11 p.223.*

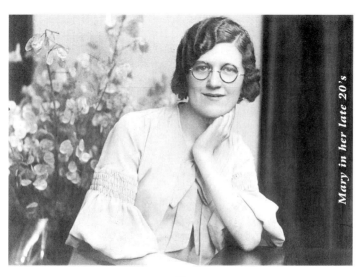

Mary in her late 20's

Conscription in the 'Private' Sector

The experience of First World War carnage was still fresh in the minds of the Government, the Services and the people. Older relatives and friends 25 years earlier, had enlisted eagerly, but now Elise and Mary shared a less excited mood, determined to walk a road of service and achievement to save the country. The partially recovered Elise told Mary that she could not face further nursing responsibilities and her over-riding horror was the possibility of hospitalisation for herself. She never lost psychological dependence on Mary and could not manage life or work apart from her. In assuming responsibility for her colleague, Mary even lost touch with her family. It was a difficult time.

Towards the end of Autumn 1941 a schoolmaster in Lancaster advertised for Christmas holiday relief in his own house, looking after his home and family. The combined expertise of the two nurses was much appreciated.

As 1942 approached conscription was biting the civilian population. Mary explained to interviewing panels [in the Civil Nursing Reserve, like the Fire Service, the Reserve was not considered as military service] that she had a dependant, so from then onwards she was conscripted into jobs where she could take Elise with her. Employers did not know that Elise was ill.

Mary's mother still working full time at the Castle Publishing Company in Preston had, together with her son Harold, taken a mortgage on a house in Thorntrees Avenue, Lea. No mortgage was then granted to a woman in her own right. In 1938 the government had appealed for volunteers for Civil Defence and Harold volunteered for the Auxiliary Fire Service, taking training in his spare time. On the day in 1939 when Germany invaded Poland he was conscripted into this service for the period of the war and became a full time fireman. Later the Auxiliary Fire Service was combined with the regular Fire Service and became the National Fire Service. These units could be sent anywhere in the area and were called to Liverpool (and elsewhere) for duty during the 'Blitz'. Harold married in 1940 and lived in Preston so the Lea house was let to a family who had left London and whose sons were in the R.A.F. Mrs. Hodkinson lived with her daughter Margaret, in rented accommodation even further out, in a cottage at Greenhalgh near Kirkham. On the 14th February 1942 she died of a heart attack and Harold had the complicated business of selling the Lea house.

The family furniture was sold. Mary's sister Margaret, working as a secretary for a timber firm on Preston Docks, found scarce lodgings and carried on doing weekend Civil Defence duty. She helped, too, in a girls' club where she was told by another helper that the now skimpy *Lancashire Daily Post* carried a notice about a bed-sitting room offered in Bells Lane, Hoghton, This was the chain of events which led Mary to Hoghton and later to Brindle in her retirement years. Hoghton became Margaret's permanent home when she moved from the bed-sitter in Bells Lane to live with Miss Anne Thompson the revered teacher of two generations of infants at St. Joseph's primary school, Brindle, who owned the next door house.

Mary looked in 1942 for another job in Lancashire and found a living-in post in a big farm house at Preston Patrick near Carnforth. The name Pumphrey was then as well known in the sugar world as Tate & Lyle now is. Mary and Elise could live as family in rooms at the farm caring for Mrs. Pumphrey senior, The Preston fox terrier, now without a home after Mrs. Hodkinson's death, was allowed to come too.

The autocratic old lady liked to issue all her instructions in the evening by pushing under her servants/nurses' bedroom door a written message that began "Mrs. Pumphrey wishes ...." One day when the pudding was taken in she pronounced "I would have preferred to have the delicious milk pudding we had yesterday." These two amateur cooks used their skilled nurses' hands to skim yesterday's rice pudding already on top of the farm dogs' bowl, but not yet put down, to wash it and re-heat it to give full satisfaction to their employer.

Family affairs now more settled and her own health restored, Mary felt free to look further afield. She was trained in the forefront of medical knowledge at the Royal Manchester Eye Hospital but the likely jobs advertised in *The Lady* magazine were to prepare her for a quite new role. She was to see out both medically and socially the financially doomed "old order" of pre-war 'England.'

The South of England presented interesting field studies in this passing. After the War's end Mary's destiny was to give practical support to survivors of the old way as they spent their declining years in great houses adapted for shared use. Later still Mary transferred her experience of the art of valiant surviving displayed in a background of gentility and good breeding to a Municipal Hospital. The art was to become a future medical specialism in which Mary was a pioneer: its new name "Geriatrics"

But in 1943, Mary was conscripted by the Civil Nursing Reserve to a private nursing home in West Sussex. Elise's housekeeping talents were used in the unique billet they shared in the village of Wivelsfield, south of Haywards Heath.

Establishments had been identified as billets (in private quarters) when war was declared, when high civilian casualties were expected. A beautiful house, Moat Cottage, was rented from the Anglican Church by Lady Carmichael where she worked under Father Salmon of East Grinstead, offering retreats Anglo-Catholic style. The Anglican Church had managed to keep control in the selection of persons billeted at Moat Cottage.

Lady Carmichael did much physical work herself but, arthritic as she was and unable to bend down, she employed a girl from the village to scrub floors. The larder had been fitted up as a little chapel and there Lady Carmichael diligently observed the Offices of the Church. One afternoon when she was at Compline, the girl, answering the front door was heard to say "No, you cannot see Lady Carmichael, she is in the chapel complaining."

The Lady had made it clear to the villagers that in Christian attitudes there must be no class distinction. The village girl shared meals at table. A tramp came to the door asking for "work". As the cottage garden was prolific with red currants and other summer fruits, including a mulberry tree so laden that it was supported by wooden props, the man was engaged to gather the harvest and clear the undergrowth. A summer house, already fitted with a bed and appurtenances for the comfort of a visitor, was offered to the tramp. When Lady Carmichael was about to accommodate him at table the girl protested "You are not going to ask that tramp? you must draw the line somewhere!"

When Lady Carmichael's lease on the cottage ran out Mary and Elise moved to rooms in Haywards Heath.

The Nursing Home in Wivelsfield where Mary worked was even more strangely managed by two unqualified ladies, sisters, by the name of Scase, who owned it. Though it was privately run, the Health Authority later intervened, placing Mary in charge. The Home was not alone in such arrangements as "buying" a patient: The proprietors of an establishment were allowed to do this, undertaking to look after a sick or old person after a certain sum was paid. There was no inspection or control.

One patient at this "Home" was the wife of a V.I.P. who had a high position in the War Office. Mary noticed that staff allocated to nursing her lasted only briefly in those duties. Only one nurse was considered by the gentleman to be compatible with the patient. It was the nurse with whom he was himself conducting a cosy little "affair".

There were old coach houses in the grounds. A ladder led up to a flat used to accommodate the mentally disabled brother of the popular historian L.du Gard Peach. His private male nurse had the misfortune to slip in icy conditions and, leg broken, was unfit for duty. Morphia was used to control the patient, but giving the injection when he was violent had never been done by any staff other than the male nurse. As the patient flailed around throwing objects, Mary mounted the ladder, syringe at the ready and told him she would stand no nonsense, and stayed until he was quiet.

Another resident, Miss Lancaster was "treated" by having her love of mice indulged. She always stayed in her room, a small piece of cheese being placed on her meal-tray for feeding to the mice. When she died, skeletons of mice were even found in jewel boxes. She was the granddaughter of the English astronomer, Sir J. F. W. Herschel who died in 1871.

One patient who was formerly a medical practitioner would lock himself in his room for three or four days.

These were civilisation's casualties. Mary's next job, though not exactly on the Front Line, gave her a glimpse of what was going on behind it.

Top Secret work with Freedom Fighters Guildford General Hospital 1944

The Civil Nursing Reserve directed Mary in 1944 to be Staff Nurse in the Casualty Department of Guildford General Hospital. Mary's job was to attend the small casualty needs of a special type of patient not allowed to associate with ordinary civil admissions. Though they were very interesting people, Mary was told not to ask questions of these "Freedom Fighters" who were trained in the mansion house in the village of Normandy west of Guildford, then dropped from aeroplanes behind enemy lines. They worked with the Free French and Free Dutch Forces. Sometimes they were able to bring escapees back to England. To overcome the language problem in hospital, a system of signals was devised. A handkerchief held in the hand in a certain way signified a broken wrist etc.

Here one was very much aware of the war. Near Guildford, the Hogs Back, a ridge of hills with hollows at the crest, became a storage place for ammunition awaiting D-Day. Before the historic announcement about landing in France residents were quietly aware that the Army was on the move.

Mary and Elise's billet was a flat in Normandy. It was large enough to welcome three children from London escaping the "doodlebugs" (Flying bombs): a girl of 7, a little boy of 4 and a scrap of a baby. The little boy had an idiosyncrasy and ate only pink food, so beetroot was used in everything. He was a bright little boy. Mary taught him to say "please" and "thank you" which he required to be used in addressing him. Mrs. Harwood, his mother, was the only parent who visited and was grateful for the care lavished on him.

The mother of the baby had been traced in Bristol. He had whooping cough, so his two nurses managed to get some wool to knit a suit warm enough for him to wear when travelling. Mary made the difficult journey by train, but though his mother did turn up at the meeting place, she said she would have nothing to do with him and departed, so Mary had to hand him into care with Bristol Social Services.

Some secret matter was troubling Elise, with serious repercussions for Mary. The only way Mary could investigate was to take to the Citizen's Advice Bureau the address in Liverpool which she had noticed written on the back of wrapping paper discarded by Elise on the coal bunker at the flat.

It was suggested that the C.A.B. should forward a message to this address. Mary wrote that she, not being a relative, was taking responsibility for Elise and asked were there not others who should do so? Mary saw no letter in reply. The C.A.B. reported that the only reply was "satisfaction that Elise was being cared for."

Elise was usually a frugal housekeeper. Mary gave her whatever cash was requested so she was amazed when the grocer could allow no more goods as the bills had not been paid. Yet there was no evidence of high expenditure on anything.

Further the manager at the local branch of the Westminster Bank reported that Elise with her large presence and commanding manner had gained access to Mary's account saying that Mary was suffering from loss of memory. Mary found that Elise had taken the drawn cash across the road to the Midland Bank and opened a new account. By her saying that regular payments would be forthcoming the Midland even granted a loan. The manager at the Westminster Bank was relieved that he was not the only one to have been fooled and he agreed to pay off the Midland, also allowing an overdraft for living expenses. Mary paid off the grocery account monthly. She was in debt to the bank and the shop to the sum of what might have been half a year's wages for people at that time. Mary never discovered where Elise has sent the money.

The rent for the flat was required and Mary's post at the Casualty Department was finishing. Would moving North solve some of these problems? Mary's sister Margaret was now sharing the home of Miss Anne Thompson, teacher of infants at St. Joseph's R.C. School, Brindle, south of Preston. Even here, between the school and the Bells Lane house, a flying bomb at Christmas, this very year, 1944, was to demolish cottages and break windows over a wide area.

One night with the sick Elise in Miss Thompson's house gave Mary time enough to realise that jobs and accommodation would be unlikely in the Preston area. She contacted Mrs. Harwood, mother of the little evacuee boy they had cared for, who offered temporary lodging in London. Mary had to accept a doctor's offer for Elise's admission to Brook Mental Hospital whilst she found private employment and rooms for herself. Mary was distressed by the quality of nursing care at the hospital (dragging patients by the hair so that the bruises would not show) and she brought Elise out after the requisite 76 hours notice.

It was at this time that Mary was given professional advice from an ex-colleague in the psychiatric field which reinforced her attitude to Elise's illness in their 46 years together.

Earlier in the Civil Nursing Reserve, Mary had worked in a unit run by Dr. Pullar-Strecker (he was a member of the Sketchley Dry Cleaning family firm) giving confidential treatment for alcoholism to very special V.I.P. politicians and Service personnel. Here there was no gentle counselling, the treatment was intense and cruel but a speedy return to full capacity was essential for the war effort. The usual treatment was by the drug Atropine to dry up body fluids.

Reluctantly Professor George Augustus Auden had come out of retirement to assist with his expertise in hypnosis, which he had used during the First World War to help shell-shocked patients. Mary herself had observed these shaking men in the streets of Preston during her girlhood. Dr. Auden had served throughout the 1914-18 war in the Royal Army Medical Corps and was the former schools' medical officer for the City of Birmingham.

Psychology and psychiatry were coming to the public attention in the 1940's and articles featured in the popular magazines. Now there was a deliberate attempt to help men when they came home on leave or were invalided out of the Services.

When Professor Auden was teaching in medical school many students had applied for tuition in hypnosis. But this gentle, thoughtful man considered it to be a highly dangerous procedure in the wrong hands. He insisted that students live in his house for six months before he decided whether to permit them to learn the full technique. He vetted their attitude to medical care, the humanities and religion before enrolling them on his course.

Many of the Servicemen who came to the unit benefited from his care and expertise. Mary thought it so sad to see these men whose broken minds and bodies had wonderfully improved, willingly go back to the same horrors they had so recently experienced.

Mary now turned for advice to the Professor whose third son Wystan Hugh Auden, an unconforming spirit, was now at this time grappling with his great poetic gifts amidst the American social scene. His father, a classicist, who had married a hospital nurse of indomitable character, was dismissive about him, disapproving of his way of life.

His experienced diagnosis of Elise's condition was that basically it would not improve and that tender loving care was the best treatment for her and that she would always require contact with Mary. Mary already knew this to be true and was already administering that care.

Mary did find work opportunities and shelter for them both. The southern counties of England had a few niches in private nursing which would suffice until the new National Health Service emerged. Some of these jobs were bizarre, feeding on the diminishing fat, the residue of Empire.

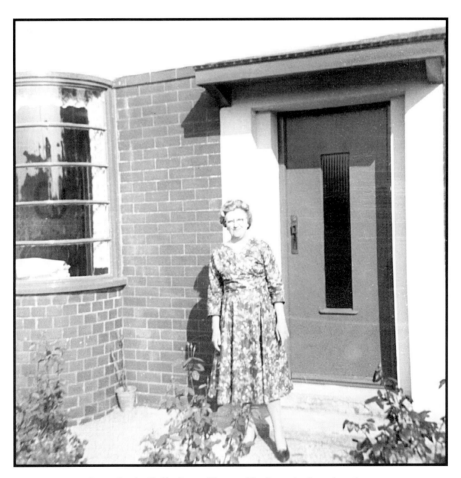

Outside the Bells Lane House, Hoghton in happier times

Survivors; an uninvaded Britain sorts itself out. 1945

A private living-in job was found in East Sussex at the village of Mayfield, notable for its variety of early architecture including the remains of a palace of the Archbishop of Canterbury. Its spectacular medieval hall had become the chapel of the Convent of the Holy Child Jesus.

Two middle aged Scottish ladies of the Kinnaird family lived in Mayfield and the war in Europe now over they resumed their enjoyment of Glyndbourne opera to which they set forth from the large family house. They be-decked themselves in the rich clothing from pre-war days and even older authentic jewels. The emeralds particularly fascinated Mary, whose taste for the theatrical had been deprived of indulgence by the grey years of war.

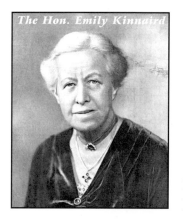
The Hon. Emily Kinnaird

As long ago as 1889 their aunt Miss Emily Kinnaird had been allocated by her parents the duty of supervising the Christian Zenana Mission in India.

In 1939, at the age of 85 she was still there handing over the management of the Mission to educated Indian women but the Second World War delayed her return to Britain In 1945, suffering from a skin condition, she came after a sea voyage, to the home of her nieces, who engaged Mary prior to her arrival to care for her. The 90 year old lady, having recovered from the disease whilst at sea, met Mary with the words "I do not need a nurse, I need a secretary. Can you write letters?"

Mary was soon writing letters from the Honourable lady to Mahatma Gandhi, addressed by her as "my dear Son" he replying to "my dear Mother." The letters discussed the setting up of a nursing care service in India.

However, assassins were closing in on both these worthy correspondents. The nieces wished to have their large house to themselves so Aunt must go to her flat in London where she had lived before the war when on furlough entertaining many student visitors from India. Her two pensioned-off maids were willing to return to care for Miss Kinnaird.

When she said "But I need Nurse, who else is there to write my letters?" the nieces replied "Letters are of no importance." In three weeks their aunt was dead.

Mahatma Gandhi was assassinated in September 1947. In 1931 he had been in London for the Round Table Conference in British-Indian Affairs. During his visit to Lancashire in August to observe the effects of his policies on the Lancashire textile industry he had stayed as guest with Blackburn people in the homes of members of the Society of Friends. So this clever barrister was, during his visit, not far away from another small valiant fighter - Mary Alicia Hodkinson.

Facsimile of a letter from Hon. Enily Kinnaird
opening the fund sponsored by many eminent people.

A frozen Winter, 1946/7. Tonsillectomy
Birmingham; Haywards Heath, West Sussex

An advertisement by two Birmingham doctors for assistance at home seemed to suit Mary and Elise's needs. Mrs.(Dr.)Wilkinson was expecting her third child and one little boy was backward in learning. After some months of the two nurses' care in the household the young boy, now nearly six, had come on well and could manage at school.

Mary closed her bank account in Birmingham and with Elise and her little terrier dog, set off back to Sussex by train. In London there was a policeman by the barrier at Victoria Station. Elise was always disturbed in crowds so travelling responsibilities were Mary's. The ticket collector said to her presenting the tickets "Have you got a little dog?" She looked round, following his glance whilst her note-case was open. Seated in the train, luggage on the rack, she realised that all the £1 and 10 shilling notes had gone from the notecase.

They were expected at lodgings with Miss Kehoe at Haywards Heath. Mary was able to secure an advance of money from her next employer. Elise found employment as cook at Crook Nursing Home.

Most survivors have vivid memories of the severe winter 1946/7. Groceries and fuel supplies(one bag of coal a week) seemed to dwindle together and ordinary life was endured rather than enjoyed.

Mary and Elise's food ration books were deposited with a grocer named Basil who lived round the corner from their lodging. This situation might have been promising: one must keep on good terms with one's grocer, the distributor of small extras. One evening Basil knocked on their lodging door for help. His father had died. Mary went with him and found the old man in rigor mortis, sitting fully dressed in a chair. His arms had been crossed against his chest and his face covered. Mary required the body to be placed on the bed in the room. Whilst she worked, Basil and the other ex-service man regaled her with their experiences in battle whilst they helped Mary to lift the body on to the bed. She was astonished by a loud scream. The fright was caused by the cover falling off its rigid face, shocking the ex-soldiers.

The association with Basil was suitably rounded off on a later occasion. He came again and asked Mary would she like to go "out". She agreed but said she must be ready for work later in the evening at Ardingly College. "Out" comprised sitting on a bench with Basil in the freezing park - so that was the end of that. The heavy falls of snow in Haywards Heath and the freezing conditions in this country generally, started on the 21st January 1947. Mary had been asked to assist Matron at the boys' school, Ardingly College. There was a 'flu epidemic and many boys were sick in this 1864 building, which has been described as "gloomy" except for its chapel.

It was a living-in job. Mary was shown to a room, given extra blankets and a hot water bottle (cold). She noticed an ancient unlit gas fire with its flue giving out from an open window,

Having survived the day's work in the old brick building with its wide stone-faced windows dripping ice and water inside and out, she decided that the train journey home was preferable to the freezing room. The college used the same link line as Lancing College and Mary worked until the Easter recess at Ardingly.

From their lodging Mary took their miniature terrier for a walk and came back feeling very ill. When she recovered from 'flu her doctor advised a tonsillectomy which was thought to be a dangerous operation. Mary agreed to undergo it if he would do it himself.

First a job must be sought. A nurse was needed at a nursing home of 15 to 29 beds in Hurstpierpoint, north of Royal Greenwich. Mary rang the doorbell here and waited. Miss Wareham, the Matron, her hands floury, answered the door. As the cook had gone, here was a job for Elise too.

Mary underwent the tonsils operation in Haywards Heath Cottage Hospital and returned to her room in the nursing home. She was working again after 5 days away. She was more or less in charge of the Home and chose to disregard the seriousness of an adult tonsillectomy.

She discovered that the Matron-proprietor's greatest joy was to manipulate people into confrontational situations and witness their disharmonious arguments.

A clever trap she set confounded all argument. One patient was a young man in his late 20's who came to the Home for a month at a time when his carers were on holiday. He suffered from disseminated sclerosis. Under the terms of some family will, Matron, Miss Wareham, was to be beneficiary if she were a married woman. Whilst his relatives were away she arranged a marriage with him, took him into her own bed in her quarters and so fulfilled the obligation of the will.

So, her financial future secured, she relinquished the Home and Mary and Elise moved on.

Individuality retained in reduced circumstances

Dane End, Hertfordshire. 1947
Dene Park, Kent. 1949

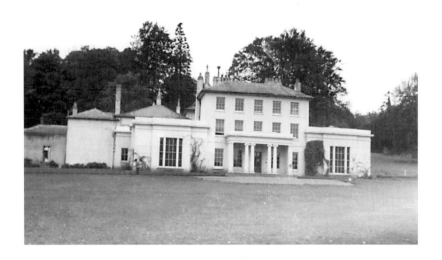

Dane End House is in a countryside estate half way between Stevenage and Ware in Hertfordshire. The ownership of this " handsome white early 19th century house of five bays and three storeys with lower side wings" (Pevsner) had, at this time, descended through the female (this due to a French connexion) line of the aristocratic Paget family, to a Mrs. Chancellor. This Paget lady was married to Mr. Christopher Chancellor who was later knighted for his work as manager of Reuters. He established a regular pheasant shoot to aid the great house's finances, and one of the participants was the writer Peter Fleming accompanied by his famous but unassuming actress wife Celia Johnson.   Mary had read his books and he remarked "that it was nice to be recognised as a writer rather than as the husband."

Mary and Elise moved in to assist Mr. Driscoll to organise the house to receive paying guests. It had become a millstone round the neck of the family and Mrs. Chancellor had been horrified by the damage inflicted on it by war-time evacuees. It was now leased to Mr. Driscoll for the Ladder League Charity of Benfleet, Surrey.

This altruistic and enterprising man had identified a need in the market for residential accommodation. The annuities of gentlefolk, after the war, in no way met, now they were deprived of servants, their expectations of refined living. One of the aims of the "Ladder Fellowship" was the provision of a care home, Dane End House.

Mrs. Chancellor, a vital woman in her 40's, moved her family - husband just back from Japan and four children - into the coachman's cottage and let the big house for a peppercorn rent. She herself set to work in the kitchen garden. The house retained the old Paget furniture. Mary remembered the Aubusson carpet in the dining room seeming more of a responsibility to her than any of the residents.

The house was equipped with four-poster beds, so Mr. Driscoll arranged for delivery of more practical furniture. Men took the first load up from the van and when they came for a second there was a woman on the tail-board speeding up the work. One man remarked to her: "They are nothing but parasites here." The woman on the tail-board heaving beds off the van was Mrs. Chancellor, parasite in chief.

The residents were an interesting bunch - all ladies. A Mr. Porter had come and gone, having tested Dane End's suitability for his needs. His presence had the effect of postponing the hour of retiring to bed as each lady strove to be the last to enjoy his exclusive company. He coped well, polite and impartial. But he went.

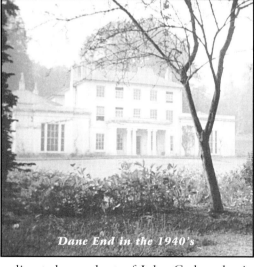
Dane End in the 1940's

One resident, Mrs. Wallace was a spirit writer. She said she was guided even by the spirits of John Milton and William Wordworth.

Another, Miss Cade, was a direct descendent of John Cade, who in 1449 led a revolt against the government. He led an army of 20,000 to place the Complaints of the Commons of Kent before the Royal Council. She had herself shared in the fight for freedom in a later century. About the year 1870 she had been with her parents in St. Petersburg where she taught the English language. When the Bolsheviks came to power she assisted a member of the British Intelligence, Paul Duke, in getting his despatches out of the country. After the murder of the Royal Family, people like Miss Cade were in danger. Mr. Duke helped her to escape via a northern port.

During the 1947-8 period Mary met Sir Paul Duke, one of the committee of the Ladder Fellowship. He was the only British Intelligence officer who had served in the Red Army. He was knighted by George V in 1936, the sole member of British Intelligence to have received this honour until the time of the second world war. Sir Paul had retained his professional technique: Mary became conscious after their encounter that he had uttered barely half a dozen words whilst she had been voluble.

Another committee member who visited was the actress Sybil Thorndike. Mary, as a schoolgirl, had seen her in Preston in 1923 when she came to speak at prize day at the Winckley Square Annexe of the Park School. When she addressed Mary at Dane End she said "I notice you have SRN behind your name. Are you connected with the Navy?"

Given the age of the residents, death and sickness were inevitable. The recessed bays of the well stocked library, out of bounds when it was a temporary 'hospital', made excellent private spaces for sick beds.

One day it was announced at breakfast that a resident's life was imminently drawing to a close. At noon Mary was approaching the entrance to the hall to sound the luncheon gong when she was surprised to see two timid ladies whose custom it was to descend the stairs for meals later than the others. "Early!" "Yes, my dear, we thought that you would not sound the gong today, not to disturb the body."

The fragments of gentility lingered on, protected after a world war which diminished a private income, by a great house and the ministrations of a northern girl whose first 'patient' was her grandmother who died in a cot at Sharoe Green one time "Workhouse" hospital at Preston. Mary had herself been gently reared and had very early in life experienced reduced circumstances, so she knew it must be harder for these older people to adjust to changes.

Few residents understood the superb contriving with food rations which made Elise's catering so interesting. Mary and Elise made a very effective team. Things were now established at Dane End, so Mary looked elsewhere.

Dene Park, Kent.

Another outlet for Mary's propensity to 'start things' was offered on an estate near Tonbridge in Kent.

Mr. Woods, like Mr. Driscoll, was a man who diligently and creatively explored the post-war market need for affordable living accommodation. With whatever modest profits he had made from film-making for the Ministry of Education during the war years, he bought in 1946 or 47 the gatehouse of a large estate, Dene Park, lived with his family there, then renovated and converted the stables into living accommodation and so sold his way on through the oast-house conversion to finding £7,000 for the mansion itself.

In the big house he began by converting its ample servants' bedrooms to private residential rooms each with a good window and open fireplace. There were 20 of these for rent to people who were unused to catering for themselves and to the unavailability of servants and old retainers,

Employed by Mr. Woods, Mary and Elise were allotted a comfortable room each. They began provisioning for cuisine and nursing care.

Downstairs from the living quarters was a large kitchen with a red quarry tiled floor. Its huge fireplace could take great logs from the park's trees. It was upgraded to being the dining room. So down the former servants' staircase soon came the paying residents dressed to honour Elise's succulent meals. The former larder had become a modern kitchen.

The large house of 1883 ('of no aesthetic merit' - Pevsner) gave comfort to those skilled in the art of gracious living, if those with the practical crafts to support it could still be found.

There was luxury too, and high life: lying next to the Dene Park Estate were the stables where the Queen's horses were trained. Social life there was struggling to re-introduce the old refinements. The stable's cook came to Dene Park to ask what sugar she should serve with coffee, Elise having acquired great status by repute in such matters.

Some of the main rooms of the mansion - one large enough for a ball-room - were later used by the Spastic Society (now re-named Scope) as a training college. During 1961-3 a purpose-built school for those suffering from cerebral palsy was erected to the east of the house.

Mary as hostess at Dene Park always met new residents at the front door. One afternoon she had been told to expect a retired lady teacher. A small car drew up outside the mansion. The lady greeted Mary but she was at pains to get "the friend who is helping me out of the back." There on the back seat covered in packages was a former influential person in Mary's life not seen for 20 years. She was Miss Stoneman, ex - Headmistress of Preston Park School for Girls who had realistically and sympathetically advised Mrs. Hodkinson about Mary's future during the Depression. She knew that this bright girl, as the eldest child of a widow with more dependants must early stand on her own feet. Now Mary was doing just that, extricating the two elderly ladies from the bundles and making them comfortable round a tea-table.

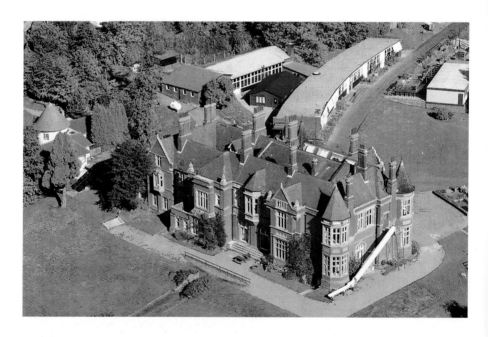

Dene Park, Tonbridge, Kent. 1949-1950
Photo: Knight Frank & Rutley - 1989
when offered for sale by the Spastics Society now renamed Scope

Ward Sister brings hope
Queen's Hospital, Croydon;
Cuckfield Hospital Sussex 1950/51

Varied activities in private nursing had been interesting and challenging but the expansion of the National Health Service was leading to more financially rewarding opportunities for qualified nurses. After the Beveridge Report leading to the National Health Service Act of 1946 the Welfare State was born.

The Festival of Britain mounted in London in 1951 expressed the national expectations of full employment. There was nationalisation of industry.

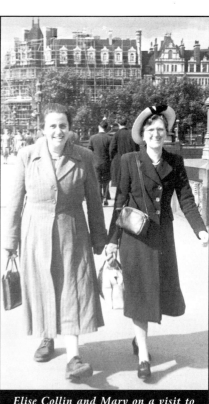

Elise Collin and Mary on a visit to the Festival of Britain, 1951

Mary looked to London. Accommodation was at a premium. Many stateless refugees, known collectively as 'foreign nationals', converged on the capital. Some were highly educated people seeking a role during the social and economic post-war turmoil and Mary and Elise met such people in a communal lodging house in Croydon. The far-sighted Mr. Driscoll known to Mary from 1947 in Hertfordshire, had adapted a terrace of Victorian houses in Addiscombe Road to basic bed-sitting rooms with fire-place and gas-ring. Each house had one bathroom for its eight rooms.

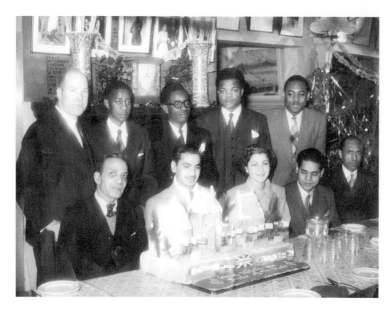

Post war unity. "Foreign Nationals"
at the International Language Club, Croydon - 1950

Named the International Language Club, admission to rent the rooms was regardless of race or creed. One day Mary opened the bathroom door to find a very tall Nigerian standing in the bath smiling down upon her and signalling a welcome.

Bishop Cuthbert of Croydon came frequently to give spiritual support. It was noticed that his visits coincided with meal times. One could opt, surrendering one's ration book and paying extra, to take meals communally in one of the houses set out on the ground floor with trestle tables and stools. Clean, well-cooked food was presented with jugs of water and bread.

Mr. Bell the chef needed help, so there was employment for Elise, who, from being unused to even boiling a single egg, could now cope with 200 served for breakfast. A stalwart worker, inspired by the handling of collective rations, Elise mixed batches of Christmas cakes and placed them in a kitchen cupboard to mature. The gradual disappearance of these precious luxuries was a puzzle until she found that there was access to the cupboard from the adjoining games room. Mr. Driscoll had been selling sixpenny slices of the stored cakes.

Mary's six month period at Croydon General Hospital in the Outpatient's Department served as a refresher course in the new drugs and treatment scene, during which time Mary and Elise found a flat in Thornton Heath.

Queen's Hospital, Croydon

She next took a post as Ward Sister at Queen's Hospital where she was responsible for 150 patients on two floors connected by a stone staircase. After the 1948 Health Act this former Workhouse Hospital was administered under central government. There was a mid-landing where the sluices and linen cupboards were, so there were numerous journeys carrying containers up and down the steps from the long "Nightingale" wards, where chronically sick people lay.

Matron at Queen's, Miss Anand was to become notable in geriatric care. At this time the study was little advanced and it was an achievement to keep patients free of bed-sores with good custodial care. But changes for the better were coming, assisted by political changes, and Mary was to be a pioneer in the field.

The postal vote for hospital patients was taken seriously at Queen's in the 1950 General Election. When the forms came each patient was approached. One, a bed-fast patient, due to her unresponsive immobility was known privately among the nursing staff as The Log. To mention of the vote she reacted like an old gun-dog. "Of course she wished to vote, had she not fought for the right as a suffragette?" She was raised from the bed and for the first time, possibly in years was dressed to make her cross on the bit of paper for which in her youth she had marched and perhaps thrown stones to gain.

One of Mary's true stories from Queen's Hospital, Croydon helps to illumine a time before affluence, mobility and reliance on "the State" has made enduring partnership of such work "alliances" as that of Mary and Elise unusual.

When this former Workhouse Hospital was brought into the NHS it was suggested tentatively (but at that time boldly) that some separated inmates formerly couples might be accommodated together in some small rooms in single beds agreed by the staff. After his partner died there, Mary was escorting the 'widower' back to the all-male ward when he remarked "We were never married. We stood together at the hiring fair, were hired together and stayed together." The Lord had provided and they saw no reason to improve on his work. Just so Mary stood with the handicapped Elise, determined to keep her promise not to desert her. No-one at this time perceived that Mary's tool, as she waited to be hired was a gun, for trouble-shooting, though this expression was yet to be coined.

Recovery from 6 years of war could in 1951 be felt. Mary's sister Margaret came from Preston to enjoy the Festival of Britain.

Mary's next move came soon after.

Cuckfield Hospital

Five miles outside Haywards Heath in West Sussex was a long stay hospital with over 200 beds for elderly people. To be nearer her new post as Ward Sister at this Cuckfield Hospital Mary moved with Elise to the village of Lindfield. A lady of good social connections, Miss Girling, possessed a timber framed house overlooking Pax Hill in the South Downs. Mary and Elise came as paying guests. They could also view the passing double decker buses, sighted through a hole in the lath and plaster wall of the bedroom.

Buses were essential. Mary caught an early one from Lindfield to Haywards Heath and completed her 10 mile journey to Cuckfield by 7.30 a.m. to start 8.0 a.m. duty, after quite a long walk to the Hospital. The night Ward Sister had a similarly difficult journey but no adjustment to rotas was countenanced by the authorities.

Other changes were under Mary's control and she set about them. Her predecessor was known to have been a 'little eccentric.' The Nissen hut wards erected for war casualties had given this earlier organiser plenty of space to separate each bed with its locker and chair so far from the next one that communication between them was impossible. Each patient lay marooned as on a raft on a sea of linoleum. Sheets were scarce, so to achieve a neat uniform military appearance the Ward Sister had arranged cut-up sheets as top flaps over the head of the blanket. They looked pristine in their whiteness. Yet some patients were lying on thick red macintosh sheets to which their skin would adhere.

Mary had permission from Matron and the visiting doctor, a G.P. from the village, to close the empty spaces so as to make the area at the bottom of the ward open for rehabilitation experiments.

With Mary had come hope, hope from complete rustication for if the patients' medical condition showed no improvement in a reasonable time their destiny was to be moved finally, further out in the countryside to The Heritage, a long stay unit managed by the Timmins family.

Many were the patients given a reprieve by Mary asking for a further 3 weeks so that together with the doctor she could reduce their drugs, change their diet, see to their mouth health (e.g. dentures) and procure spectacles after eyesight tests. The Hospital Secretary said what a difference the progress in this ward had made to the whole hospital.

At this time publications on gerontology were appearing on both sides of the Atlantic; job descriptions in the Health Service in Britain began to reflect the interest.

Mary noticed in the *Nursing Mirror* an advertisement for a Matron responsible for admission and care of older people from an acute hospital to a unit to be established near Leeds for rehabilitation. She remarked to Elise "I wonder what sort of damn fool they'll give this job to?" The challenging reply was "Why don't you apply and find out?" Mary took up the challenge.

More scope for a pioneer; Matron wins male equality

Haigh Hospital, Rothwell, Leeds. 1952-54.
W.H.O. Seminar and Ninth World Health Assembly

After a very tedious Sunday journey by train to Leeds, Mary found a taxi. The telegram had directed her to attend for interview at Seacroft Hospital. At 3.0 a.m., the driver thought there would be a more ready reception at Killingbeck Hospital and sure enough a helpful domestic got permission from Matron, via Night Sister's office, for Mary to be accommodated there until the interview.

After a few hours' sleep she was taken to Matron's office at 7.45 a.m. where a corner of a table was laid for breakfast. Matron made an entrance, her large cloak flurrying behind her, and delivered her judgement on the encroaching bureaucracy and Mary's prospects within it. "They don't want MATRONS any more, they only want Yes-people. It's no good for you here."

Mary thought differently. She was selected, gave one month's notice at Cuckfield, and moved in to work under Group B Management Committee of Leeds which was based on Seacroft Hospital: (St. James' - used in the T.V. programme *Jimmy's* was in Group A).

A vacated former isolation hospital The Haigh was to be set up to house the rehabilitation unit. A small domestic staff had been retained. Mary was now experienced enough to enjoy exploiting the opportunities for engaging new staff. A born administrator of a human institution she knew that this power was crucial to smooth achievement.

A new Secretary had been appointed to the executive Hospital Management Committee, a Mr. Brown, well used to command as a former Flight Lieutenant in the R.A.F. Mary found the committee members to whom she reported monthly, a very supportive team. Some were private employers, some representatives of trade unions and charities. Their appointment by the Health Service, via the Regional Health Authority who submitted names of likely persons, aimed to secure a balance to serve the five or six hospitals in the community of Leeds, the lively centre of commerce and industry.

Mr. Brown had found a good clerk of works and supplies officer and Mary knew where she stood with regard to the administration. A joiner or plumber would arrive with a job form showing expected time of arrival and departure which Mary signed. The clerk of works came to check the work done.

The supplies officer, Mr. Lord, ensured that perishable and durables arrived according to need when Mary submitted her orders to the supplies office. Mr. Lord had high standards. He requested that the new Matron accompany him to buy household furnishings for her quarters, which he estimated would require nice linen and a complete 12 cover dinner service; 12 sherry and champagne glasses would be the minimum and these were duly packed. A remark was passed that this was not a National Health order but a private purchase by Matron herself.

After Mary's subsequent moves all that remain are a few sherry glasses and one tureen. These British made articles had more than earned their keep by oiling working relationships at inter-hospital entertainments and helping Mary to ease-in ideas for the rehabilitation of her patients. That was the primary aim.

The hospital building comprised an administration block, Matron's quarters and the usual male and female wards. At the bottom of the drive stood a large wooden building with a verandah looking out over fields. It was in good condition so Mary made it attractive as a Day Room. To reach it patients had to don good shoes, coat, hat and gloves. Forty or fifty people could go there leaving thoughts of illness behind them.

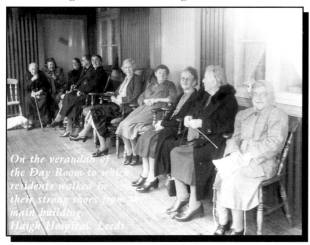

On the verandah of the Day Room to which residents walked in their strong shoes from the main building Haigh Hospital, Leeds

In a nearby community, an over 60's Club had been established. On Thursdays a bus took some of the patients there, if necessary accompanied by a member of staff. If there was some special birthday the 'host' or 'hostess' could welcome two or three guests from the club back to the rehabilitation unit to an informal party where they were seated at the top of the table. This was an area of treatment where smaller numbers and social interaction in a pleasant environment achieved best results. 70th birthdays were celebrated as a wonderful milestone reached.

The first TV set at The Haigh was secured for the Day Room in time for the Coronation of Elizabeth II on 2nd June 1953. Mary organised the viewing with a remembrance of her own street visit to an earlier Coronation. Each patient, ready in hat and coat, took a special packed lunch to the Day Room, walking down the drive for an uninterrupted entertainment and celebration with hot drinks to hand.

Many patients were former wool-workers suffering from chest conditions; also from malnutrition, due to ignorance of good feeding habits. An excellent cuisine had been assured by Mary appointing Elise as cook. Since she was self-trained during war conditions, she had no quantities or ingredients from an era of affluence to forget. Resourceful with rations, inventive, living with her nose in a cookery book, she had a reputation for achieving excellence at economical rates. Indeed, Mary received her only reprimand in her administrative career in that her catering costs were too low.

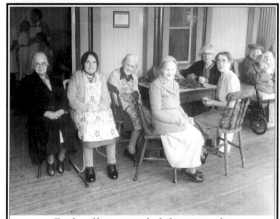

Early efforts at rehabilitation, the Day Room at Haigh Hospital. A resident cradles in his arms John William's (assistant matron) Yorkshire Terrier.

Elise could work best alone so although the kitchen closed for main meals at 5.30 p.m. Elise would go back to prepare for the following day. If the night porter saw that she had reached the clearing-up stage at 2 a.m. he knew the light would soon be out.

Another valuable appointment was an ex-ship's steward who applied for the position of gardener. He had no qualifications for this but had been advised after his de-mobilisation Navy medical examination to get an outdoor job to assist recovery from T.B.. He had been engaged on the ship that took King George VI, Queen Elizabeth and the Princesses to Canada on their first overseas trip after the Coronation. His experience there in mixing special cocktails more potent than usual (and for which he would not divulge the recipe) gave Mary a special power over the management committee.

The Chairman of the committee, Mr. Brooks, had the duty of looking in for a half hour at the Christmas parties in each hospital, these events being held usually on the same evening. He arrived at the beginning of his duty trek at The Haigh first of all and demanded a gin, saying "he was already miserable at the prospect and might as well get worse." But Elise's buffet and the gardener-steward's provision cheered him up so much that he never arrived at the other hospitals. Next morning he paid a more formal call to the office and said he had not known what it was all about last night but he had enjoyed himself. A young nurse replied "Yes you did enjoy it - you kissed Matron!"

The question of a deputy for Matron was discussed. Throughout all the period of time establishing new procedures Mary had felt that she could take no time away from the hospital.

Opportunities were occurring for men in nursing. The Ministry of Health was offering crash courses to medical orderlies, particularly those with experience in military hospitals, to become SRN's, and these had now made their way into general hospitals.

Mary's proposal that a male nurse should be sought for the position as Deputy was accepted by the Committee on the clear understanding that should this appointment, regarded as an experiment fail, Mary would shoulder total responsibility. Out of the many mixed applications three candidates were selected for interview and Arthur Williams, a Navy-trained nurse, was appointed as Assistant Matron.

Arthur brought his wife, child and a Yorkshire terrier, which slept on the desk, in the in-tray. His master, a 6-footer, swapped him for Mary's Samoyed named Happy when going for walks. Arthur and Mary worked

together with such dove-tailed efficiency that further stimulus was looked for.

Financially it would not impair Mary's career if she looked for another post, whereas Arthur's position, with a wife and small child resident in the grounds and no appointment beyond

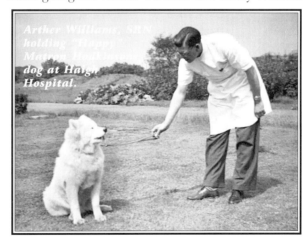

Arthur Williams, SRN holding "Happy", Matron Northcote's dog at Haigh Hospital.

Charge Nurse in general nursing being allowed to him, was less flexible.

This led to a discussion relating to the position of male and female staff in the Health Service. The College of Nursing, the Regional Council and the Regional Nursing Officer were approached for the views on the appointment of a male nurse to the senior position of Matron.

Many senior nurses who accepted that a male patient could be nursed by a female nurse could not reconcile themselves to the reverse. All the answers to the questionnaire were returned in the negative.

Arthur was very disappointed at this result. There was only one authority further to which Mary could apply. She drafted a letter to the late Ian McLeod, Minister of State for Health, pointing out that the influx of male nurses to the NHS and their extended training led to economic waste, if, proceeding through the present training system, these candidates were not allowed to reach the top positions, It was also morally wrong.

A correspondence led to the Minister conceding the proposals and authorising the Management Committee to consider appointing Mr. Williams, subject to the appointment vote being unanimous.

The Secretary of the Ministry of Health at Savile Row, London, W.1. wrote on the 20th August, 1954.

Dear Madam,

I have been asked to write and thank you for your letter of the 28th July, about the appointment of male nurses to the position of Matron.

The Minister, was glad to have the information you have given and, in coming to a decision on the appointment of a Matron at the Haigh Hospital, he has taken into account the views expressed in your letter.

Yours faithfully,
S. W. Jamieson.

So Arthur Williams became Chief Nursing Officer, the first male Matron ever appointed. Mary applied for a post in Jersey.

World Health Assembly, Geneva 1954 and 1956

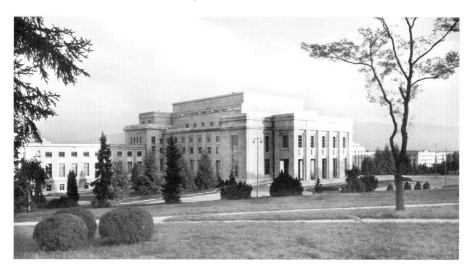

The Jersey post under the States Greffe was one in which Mary would need to be able to stand back from the chaotic social and political scenes being enacted on the off-shore island. She spent two weeks of her summer break from Haigh Hospital on a study course that gave a world perspective on the health scene. It was held in Geneva.

There was a further reason why Mary chose a working holiday. She knew that Elise Collin's fragile emotional health might erupt in the anger and incomprehension an infant feels on the withdrawal of care. The risk of taking the sort of holiday with other significant relationships perceived by Elise as a threat, might rock the boat of Mary's vocational fulfilment balanced on the sea of a 14 year old promise and the tender loving care advocated by Professor Auden as the only treatment for her colleague's disability.

In March 1954 a notice in the *Nursing Mirror* offered places on the 6th Seminar organised by the World Health Organisation, where a wide range of health problems would be covered in exercises known as technical discussions. Applicants would be required to finance themselves entirely, suitable guest houses being identified.

The theme of this seminar was "Nurse training and the nurse's role in the health team". The lecturers were professors, experts in their own field of leprosy, malaria, alcoholism etc.

The representatives from many developing countries had had very little experience of nursing as known in the western world but were very eager to learn how to set up health services for their own people. Europe was also in turmoil with many refugees and stateless persons who had to be 'processed'. Mr. Ennals, now Lord Ennals, was at that time the W.H.O. Commissioner for Refugees. He did heroic work for these people in a very tiny office in Geneva.

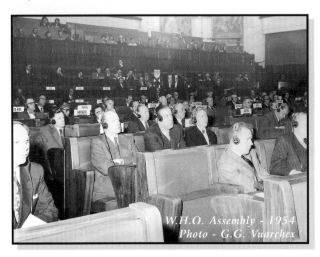

W.H.O. Assembly - 1954
Photo - G.G. Vuarchex

Seminar lectures were in the morning; the plenary sessions of the technical discussions followed in the afternoon. They had been held in individual groups and were based on the reports received from about 55 government members of W.H.O. So though on the same theme, these latter were more politically biased.

The cultural differences between these 'civilised' delegates were high-lighted in the Swiss boarding house where Mary stayed with other female colleagues. The lavatory was positioned at the far end of an open games room. A visit there included the unwelcome courtesy and heel-clicking of some delegates, Prussian doctors who bowed one in, opening the lavatory door helpfully.

In the 1956 study course, discussions on world health themes were to be drawn to a conclusion. Though there were no seminars Mary asked if she could be present as an observer, She made a second visit to Geneva to the Ninth World Health Assembly. Papers dealt comprehensively with nursing education. There were now government delegates from 88 countries.

Representing Britain were Sir John Charles, Minister of Health, and his team, also Dame Elizabeth Cockayne D.S.E. Chief Nursing Officer within the Ministry of Health and recently appointed Chief Nursing Officer of W.H.O. In that position she was chairman of all the plenary sessions. She was succeeded in 1956 by Miss Creelman from U.S.A.

There were many world political figures in Geneva at a conference sorting out the problems of North and South Korea. They met at the Palais de Nations, occupying the lion's share of it.   The W.H.O. people had to have special passes to be admitted to their allocated corner. The Soviet delegates to the conference were very wary and vetoed the W.H.O. from holding its dance in the marble hall of the Palais.

Mary witnessed the arrival of V. M. Molotov, General Secretary of the Supreme Soviet, a little figure deposited under the portico of the Palais de Nations. All the curtains of his car were drawn and the vehicle itself was protected on all sides by six Cadillacs. Out of each vehicle six Cossacks stepped.   The cavalcade was waiting to receive the U.S.S.R. statesman after the meetings.

Sir Anthony Eden, British Foreign Secretary, was called for by a girl driver in a small saloon car into which he lowered himself without ceremony and it nipped away easily through the traffic. Britain's contribution to the party-giving was similarly inconspicuous: there were many small receptions sponsored by the various countries, none by Britain.

When the dance was held, Mary had an opportunity to identify these low-profile Britons. Lacking the marble hall of the Palais, the dance was held in two adjacent hotels at the side of the lake in the centre of Geneva, Dr. Kaplan (USA) organising it and receiving the guests. Each lady was presented with a carnation and a car-key case with WHO, Geneva, 1956 emblazoned on it in gold.

Mary enjoyed herself recognising guests from the 1954 Seminar, gathered round the tables chatting. Noticing the British delegation standing stiffly in a further part of the room she determined to seek them out.

The strict clothes rationing of that time had not allowed Mary the security of entirely suitable dancing shoes and as she crossed the polished floor her foot slipped and she fell in a heap in front of the delegation, announcing "I am from the United Kingdom." After being escorted solicitously back to her seat to enjoy the Folie Bergeres and the Dance of the Seven Veils, Mary was approached by Sir John Charles for a dance on the absurdly small floor where one could only wriggle. She noticed that the Britons, their feet rather than their tongues in action, wriggled rather more enthusiastically than anyone.

Neatly filed for future reference, Mary retained all the World Health Organisation papers distributed at the two conferences. At that time 24% of the W.H.O. were nurses, so their expertise was well represented. Items in the 1956 W.H.O. Newsletter read as if written in the 1990's : "The nurses .... are loaded with so much additional work that they complain they cannot adequately care for their patients." "The amount of time to be given to each patient in regard to tests, checks and records etc. has increased." "In the pressure of work due to scientific progress the immediate physical needs of the patient are attended to but the emotional and humane ones may be overlooked."

Quoted from a British report in the heading of the 1956 Newsletter "It is difficult to say if modern changes are good or bad .... but the mental trauma of being apparently treated as a scientific experiment rather than a sick individual is at times evident."

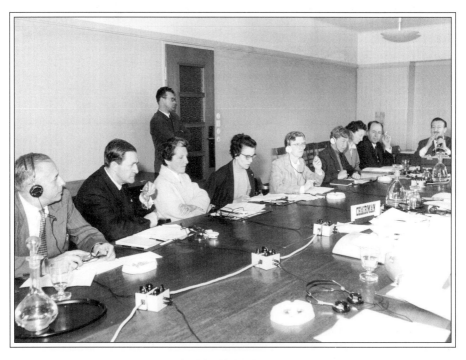

W.H.O. Assembly 1956. Discussion Group.
Mary 5th from the left. Photo: J.G. Cadoux.

Sorting off-shore sleaze
Sandybrook Hospital, St. Peter, Jersey. 1954-1955

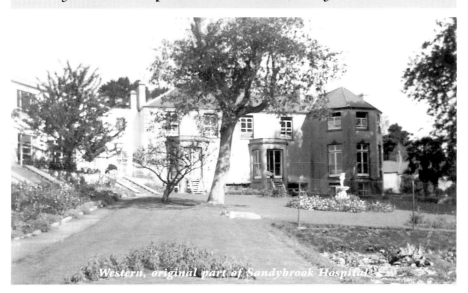

Western, original part of Sandybrook Hospital

During the Nazi occupation of the Island of Jersey, senior hospital staff had struggled valiantly to continue a system of training for girl entrants to the nursing profession. There could be no substitute for specialist training on the mainland which formerly comprised an important part of the course. The three main island hospitals had to suffice for experience.

When Mary was appointed as Matron to Sandybrook Hospital at St. Peter's Bay with a particular brief to sort things out there it was nine years after the Second World War's end. Still a shaky administration made repercussions throughout the island.

Her task of re-organisation was not assisted by the quality of the staff attracted, after deprivations and scarcities, to a comparatively sybaritic life. While salaries in the public sector were the same rate as on the mainland, here there was low income tax and no purchase tax. Goods brought by international shipping were available in luxurious variety. The acquisition and enjoyment of these, the pleasant climate and the opportunity to find a rich husband in commerce, had made staff nurse posts a magnet for S.R.N's. from the mainland.

Sandybrook had its share of these. There was also a skeleton staff of more dedicated Gervaise, many quite unqualified. So that rooms in their families' homes could be lucratively let to visitors to the island, a good number of these elected to live-in at the Hospital.

In this holiday-camp background Mary found haphazard staffing arrangements without settled ward routines. Nursing standards were poor. She noticed one assistant washing the hands and faces of five patients without changing the water.

Mary had had to serve three months notice in her Leeds post, so whilst she was awaited at Jersey to replace the dismissed Matron, a local Ward Sister was temporarily in charge. She was a lady in her 30's, serious, conservative, and efficient. Mary recognised her as a delightful person to work with. She had had an impossible role in relation to the go-getting S.R.N's from the mainland who would dominate her and continue their habit, acquired under the sloppy regime of the alcoholic ex-matron, of ordering a packed lunch from the kitchen and disappearing to the beach, leaving poor Ward Sister to carry on.

Her shaky confidence in herself had been further undermined in encountering her own record in the personnel file when she was doing the ex-matron's office work. She was considered to be an "average nurse but not a person who could be allowed to manage on her own initiative." Mary reassured her and knew she was just the dependable person she needed.

A problem that was easily sorted out was an area of gross neglect, with regard to a dozen or so girl 'patients' who lived in a small building apart from the hospital, and who were supposed to look after themselves with complete freedom of movement and coming to the refectory for meals. Sandybrook was a hospital for old people but these girls might be suffering from mild epilepsy, low I.Q. or were regarded as 'subnormal'.

Their existence was scarcely recognised, though linen was dumped to them now and then. Without supervision their rooms were in an appalling state. Mary found mouldy sandwiches under mattresses and even a half opened tin of sardines.

Mary ensured that care of the girls should be brought under hospital services and some were admitted to the wards as patients. There was no difficulty in ordering and providing of suitable clothing for them from the Social Services.

Establishing efficient ward administration required a measure of ruthless courage which Mary possessed, but, in achieving order, her direct style and compromising boldness in dealing with powerful political undercurrents cost her her job.

The Matron of nearby St. Helier's Hospital delivered her own verdict: "This need not have happened. You have been a fool. You chose to sleep in the wrong bed." She spoke as a practical woman used to the accepted French culture of le menage a trois or la maitresse.

To achieve her aim Mary had used power that did not exist in a similar position on the mainland where she would have been responsible to a Hospital Management Committee. Under the Jersey system, responsible directly to the Minister of State, she could appoint and dismiss staff at will.

One evening, for every member of her staff, juniors, cooks and all nurses, she typed out and circulated a notice to quit. A new contract, devised by Mary, could be signed by staff at Matron's office on Monday morning.

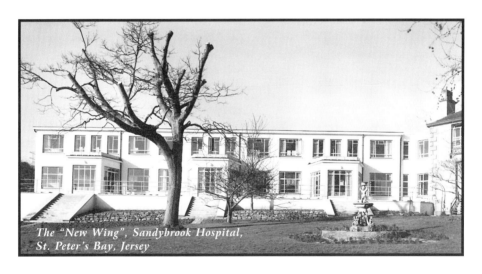

The "New Wing", Sandybrook Hospital, St. Peter's Bay, Jersey

Nurses from the mainland whose aims were material and social rather than professional refused to sign. There remained a skeleton staff of 12 sympathetic nurses to serve 100 patients. Mary advertised vacant posts and it was not long before journalists from the *Jersey Sun* and the politicians were exploiting the now public situation.

The Senators of the Jersey Parliament each held office as Ministers of State. The man who had held the office of President just prior to Mary's arrival was Mr. Le Marquand. He was alleged to have had a more than a professional relationship with the previous Matron of Sandybrook. At the General Election of early 1954 he lost his seat and the problem of Matron's weakness for alcohol was left to his successor, Mr. T. G. Le Marinel. Now responsible for the hospital he was eager to improve its status and had appointed Mary as new Matron.

When Mary was making the necessary changes, preparations for the next election were looming and the unpopular staff-improvement moves fell handy for exploitation by politicians. The journalists had a field day. Mr. Le Marquard, to manipulate opinion in the Senate in readiness to get back into power, came into the hospital wards. He went from bed to bed interviewing patients in the Gervaise language and later issued garbled statements that the patients had had "nothing to eat to-day" or were "suffering from lack of attention." Mary had to attend unpleasant interrogative meetings with the Hospital Committee relating to these fabrications.

During this ferment the remaining dedicated staff ran the Hospital in increasingly good order. The Ward Sister who had filled the post of Matron during the interregnum before Mary's arrival went away sick for two months. Mary, who knew her capabilities, was determined to support her. With the agreement of the Steward-General of all the Jersey Hospitals she made personal visits to her home to give her confidence by arranging and offering working hours of her own choice. "Yes, she would arrive at 10.0 a.m. next Monday morning."

The nurse's brother, friendly in his relations with Mary, came instead at 8.0 a.m. to report the tragic news that she had hanged herself.

A new Ward Sister was appointed from the mainland. At first she managed very well but then developed delusions that people were chasing her. Mary had a problem here as mental illness as such was not recognised in the Jersey system. One had to be labelled "mad" to go to St. Ocan's, labelled "sick" to go to St. Helier's or "old" to be admitted to Sandybrook. Mary had the Sister's condition diagnosed as physical so that she could be admitted to Sandybrook sick bay.

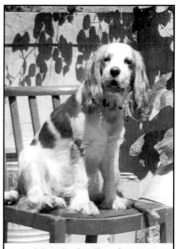

Mary's dog Powder at Sandybrook Hospital, Jersey.

However, her return to the mainland seemed to be the only practical course. The airline required that a nurse should see the patient onto the plane. At the Hospital entrance all was packed ready but when the taxi drew up the Ward Sister dashed to it and went, leaving Mary behind. Another taxi had to be ordered and a chase made to ensure that she boarded in good order.

During this time Elise had earned a small salary looking after Matron's quarters. Soon she and Mary were boarding a plane too to leave the Island, the Senate having unanimously agreed Mary's resignation.

Mary's Hospital Report 23rd August 1954 to October 1955, (Number of patients 101), comprises nine long sheets of close typing with not a wasted word, outlining the gradual re-organisation of the institution which had got by on patient labour, even of the unsupervised mentally defective residents, performing such tasks as lighting and fuelling the coke boiler and inefficiently washing crockery; then preparing food in uncleaned rooms and passed it to a cook who resented any interference in her routine. Drugs in the cupboard did not tally with the book, open commodes were left at strategic points. Soiled linen was left on the floor. It was assumed that night staff washed the patients, but this in fact was not carried out; there was delay in distributing 32 dinners stacked on plates in a lift, top floor patients' meals were carried up two flights of stairs; cleanliness generally was of a low standard. Washing water was not changed even between attending to incontinent patients. Domestic staff helped with patient care as there were too few nurses.

In Mary's account of the overhaul of domestic conditions, professional staffing and secretarial administration, her paragraph on services includes as well as medical and chaplain visits, the library service by the Red Cross. "The addition of children's books for the mentally defective patients has been a successful innovation. St. John's Ambulance Cadets maintained a steady flow of voluntary workers. The Salvation Army band comes every quarter to play on the terrace."

The crowning achievement at the receiving end was that "bed ridden patients have been got up and now enjoy friendly chats with other patients. Two hemiplegic patients have been taught to walk again. All this is spite of the lack of a physiotherapist." and "Mentally defective patients have been made to feel they are of importance." Each patient was equipped with three sets of clothing marked for their own use. Mary accompanied her report with a letter to the President and Public Health Committee:

> *Dear Sirs,*
>
> *I herewith submit a Hospital Report on the past fourteen months. Whilst every effort has been made to condense it to reasonable proportions it has been necessary to write a fairly comprehensive one, owing to the amount of structural alterations and general re-organisation that has taken place. I should like to acknowledge indebtedness to Dr. Clyde, the Steward General, and all my staff for the help and support they have given me. Without their aid it would have been impossible to put Sandybrook Hospital on such a firm foundation.*
>
> *I wish Miss Owen every success and happiness in her new position.*
>
> *Yours faithfully,*
> *Matron.*

On Saturday 17th September 1955 The *Jersey Sun* quoted as usual a SAYING OF THE WEEK. Chap. VI. verse 4 from Ecclesiastes was chosen. "For he cometh in with vanity and departeth in darkness." Underneath it was a short news item -"Sandybrook Matron to go" which affords a classic example of journalistic muddle: " She is to be replaced by the present Assistant Matron [correctly Miss Owen] Miss M. A. Hodkinson."

On the 24th October 1955 Mary received a letter from the Greffier of the States thanking her and that "despite the difficulties which you encountered at the commencement of your appointment the Committee feels that you have succeeded in bringing about an increased measure of discipline and order in the administration of the hospital.", and signing himself "Your obedient servant."

It was a position few could have achieved. Mary was grateful for the support she had received from the Royal College of Nursing who had taken a serious view of the whole situation.

Mary had no regrets: she had performed the task, but the age of the professional trouble-shooter had not yet arrived.

A vision of the future in a resistant, crumbling world

Tolmers Park Hospital, Hatfield, Hertfordshire. 1955-7

Mary was appointed as resident Matron in December 1955 in a hospital for old people under the North London Management Committee whose responsibility included The Royal Free Hospital and The Prince of Wales Hospital.

Tolmers Park, with under 100 patients, was in the village of Newgate Street near Cuffley, Hertfordshire. This old house now drawn into the N.H.S. was once in the ownership of the Earl of Salisbury and it had been sympathetically converted to hospital use. There was a delightful semi-circular part from which wards radiated making very pleasant areas.

As the building was only two miles away from the Jacobean Hatfield House it was reputed to have been the home of Arabella Stuart, who secretly married the Marquis of Hertford and so alienated Charles 11. There was the tradition that the couple had been imprisoned in Tolmers.

The arrival of the two ladies from the North - Mary and Elise- seemed to set the old house crumbling. An Adams fireplace which graced the room allocated to Elise collapsed onto the floor. The clearing of old laurel bushes which surrounded the house was followed during the night by another collapse resulting in a crater which was found to lead to a crypt. This was made safe and left open as a garden feature.

Other achievements dependent upon mere human urgency and energy were slow to start. The Hospital Secretary was a Mr. Grey who always wore grey suits. He did at last order the re-fixing of the kitchen sinks which were held to the wall with rags. Their nooks made a cosy breeding ground for cockroaches which hung nose to tail on the walls.

Mary had had similar cockroach trouble at Jersey. There, the French cook insisted on the walls being washed down each morning after the nightly cockroach visitation. Mary at last achieved re-fixing and there was a final swilling down in which she summoned her schoolgirl French to compare it to "La mer" whilst the cook pointed to the last black "poisson" floating away in disinfectant.

At Tolmers too, many of the staff were from the European mainland. There was a Lithuanian married couple and Spanish and Italian girls who had been internees in nearby camps during the war. So Mary got used to being addressed as "Mama mia" by two kitchen girls who had mastered the phrase "me not understand" to evade unwelcome tasks.

When one of the Spanish girls was caught shop-lifting in Marks & Spencers in Enfield Mary went to Court as a character witness to support her. Stores were changing from behind-the-counter drawers to open display of goods and this was one of the first. The girl stated that she had assumed that goods lying about were for picking up. Mary found a selection of items in the girl's bedroom so they were able to be returned in their cellophane wraps. The most embarrassed person in court was the young male trainee who had caught her. Everything had to be translated including the re-enactment of holding of bra and pants against her body to test the size, an action not much aired in public in the 1950's. If the "foreign nationals" sent money home, the amount, was exempt from British income tax.

As there was a settled nursing staff it was necessary to replace only one Ward Sister. Mary began a rehabilitation programme. Patients were dressed and left their beds for the day room. Male nurses came from other hospitals in the management area and assisted with the lifting in the female wards. All seemed to be going well.

Hospitals were still allowing voluntary helpers under the scheme remaining from the war era when labour was scarce. Some" county ladies" came *when* they wished and did only *what* they wished. Resistance to change came from this quarter. One of these occasional ladies found out that some patients, well on the way in the rehabilitation process, were being taken home for visits by supportive relatives eager to advance recovery. She found that Mary had not asked for the necessary permission and organised formal complaints.

A complaint about a male nurse came from another "volunteer" making much of a remark passed by a patient in the female ward. Sister on duty had seen nothing wrong in asking an excellent young male nurse to assist in the ward at night when a patient had an "accident ". He was a sunny natured person dedicated to service. He had uttered the reassuring pleasantry "Don't worry, we'll soon have you looking like Marilyn Monroe." Another patient resented his remark, reporting that he was "doing it for his own gratification." The volunteer made an issue of this, yet it had been officially agreed that male nurses should be brought into female wards particularly assisting with lifting but subject to certain restrictions.

Geriatric Care Association

Such pettiness did not blur Mary's vision of the future. It was at Tolmers in 1956 that she suggested to the profession the formation of a geriatric Nurses Association. It was cold shouldered.

Post Graduate Course on Geriatric Nursing

She also outlined a procedure and curriculum with a very practical component based on a job assignment basis at the hospital, which itself with its new nurses home, in beautiful gardens set in wooded countryside and social and educational opportunities in nearby London, would attract the well-motivated student nurse.

However, the unsettled atmosphere aggravated Elise's nervous condition. Her comments about the hospital policy whilst working in the hospital kitchen led the Secretary to ask for her removal. Mary found her a live-in housekeeper job at Fisk's drapers in St. Albans. She gave satisfaction but, her health deteriorating, she was unable to cope. Her next job was a living-in post at Grendon T.B. Hospital as cook.

But she could not, away from Mary, stay on an even keel. There was a distressing "self-protecting" reaction by Elise when Mary chatted about a new interesting man friend, a contact in the hospital administration, whose company Mary had been enjoying. The uncontrollable rage with which this information was greeted was similar to that manifested by those suffering from untreated post-traumatic stress disorder, recognised as an illness only 30 years later.

With a soldier-nurse's fortitude Mary picked up the laden stretcher and carried on. She herself must face changes. The Matron of the Royal Free Hospital had intimated that the Management Committee considered that the methods of treatment at Tolmers were not what they wanted. So having served 2 years Mary gave 3 months notice. She was to go to Peterborough.

Elise had found excuses to be dissatisfied with her job at Grendon Hospital. There was a prison nearby and she claimed that there had been intruders in her room. She put pressure on Mary to be allowed to join her in the nice first floor flat in Lincoln Road, Peterborough.

Mary found Elise a job as a live-in housekeeper to the Bishop of Peterborough. Here she developed serious leg problems and could not stand. After being admitted to hospital in late summer 1957 for an operation, until March 1988 when she died in Lancashire, she was formally recognised as an invalid , an invalid in Mary's private care.

The King Charles spaniel, Powder, who had come back with them from Jersey was upset by all the changes. One morning when in charge of the landlady at the flat she ran out and was killed by a bus.

Centralisation; stupid routines on the wards cleared
St. John's Hospital, Peterborough 1957-1959

Mary had answered an advertisement for an Assistant Matron in charge of a satellite hospital of Peterborough Memorial Hospital. It was housed in the former St. John's Workhouse Hospital, all under the same Management Committee.

The retiring Matron of St. John's had been used to saving pennies and making up stereotype medicines - castor oil, syrup of figs, cough mixture etc. Bottles were rinsed out and re-used. She also dispensed disinfectants. A "cough mixture" bottle was used for pure lysol and sent to the ward. A dose of this administered to a patient resulted in death.

The Matron of Peterborough Memorial Hospital used this inefficiency to support a centralization plan, which improved her own status. It was agreed that the Orthopaedic, Fever and St. John's Hospital, be drawn together under this Miss Richards, Assistant Matrons being in charge of the others.

Mary had already been acquainted with the long wards of "the workhouse" at Queen's Hospital, Croydon, but the antiquated routine at St. John's she could not accept. Facilities were minimal. There was the Assistant Matron's office central to the wards. Next to that was a staff locker room and toilet facilities. All the patients were "bed-fast."

It was a very long established custom that, after breakfast was served to the 40 or so patients, the nursing staff started at the right hand side of the landing from the office and proceeded attending to the patients in strict sequence. Those first attended to were, not surprisingly, the only residents without the label "incontinent."

Mary ordered that all should have prompt toilet facilities. But an automatically performed routine could not be broken by a reasonable order. So Mary pocketed the key to the staff toilet. She noticed frequent visits to the locked door. It was nearly time for lunch when Mary was approached by one of the nurses in desperation. She produced the key from her pocket having made the point that in future every patient should have this personal basic right. It was the nurses' first lesson in the rehabilitation of the elderly. The ward orderlies saw the funny side of Mary's plot, and all worked well together.

Dr. Walker was the Senior Physician of the Memorial Hospital. He had the authoritative flamboyance of Professor Lancelot Spratt of Richard Gordons' *Doctor in the House* published in 1952. On one occasion, when there was a possible outbreak of food poisoning, he arrived in the ward with a two litre bottle of Kaolin and morphine mixture - the usual medicine for this at that time. All patients were to be dosed with it. He said it was a way of counter-balancing likely press reports, and he told Mary that he would have preferred to be a journalist.

Mary remarked to him that the new antibiotics and other drugs now in use to combat infections would save much surgery. He made the prophetic reply (it was 1957/8) that surgeons would never surrender their position of superiority and mystery, and it would not be long before they were looking at spare parts.

The Assistant Matrons met each other for the first time months after Mary was in post. They were summoned to Miss Richards' office after lunch for coffee where Mary was the recipient of their sympathy. All agreed that Miss Richards (she ran an Austin 7) was not making the satellite hospitals regular visits as was expected - though St. John's Geriatric, the nearest, saw her occasionally.

There was also vacillation by the Management Committee. Some members , those from Trade Unions, were appointed, not elected. The local authority was responsible for St. John's Hospital, but the Management Committee had over-all charge of the Peterborough hospitals. When they got back to their own councils some members of the H.M.C's vetoed what they had agreed at the Management Committee. These two-faced tactics had the result that the extension to Peterborough Memorial Hospital took seven years to be agreed.

One day Mary was asked by Miss Richards' deputy , Miss Hulme, if she knew anything about senior staff resigning their posts. Miss Richards was pushing for this and Miss Hulme herself was going as Matron to Wolverhampton General Hospital. Sure enough, Mary was summoned to the office by Matron Richards, thanked for her work at St. John's and told that after two years it was time to move.

At last: scope to bring abundant life
Catmose Vale Hospital, Oakham,
Rutland 1959-1968

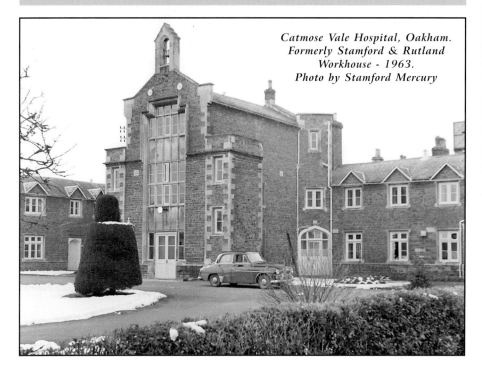

Catmose Vale Hospital, Oakham.
Formerly Stamford & Rutland
Workhouse - 1963.
Photo by Stamford Mercury

Mary was prodded to her next move by Matron Richards at Peterborough: "have you done anything about that cat and mouse Hospital?" She was referring to Mary's mentioning an advertised vacancy under Sheffield Regional Hospital Board, for a Matron to take charge of the elderly and chronic sick at Catmose Vale, Oakham.

What better time to attend for an interview and to have a choice before one than in late April, when the rural background bloomed welcome? When Mary left the railway station at Oakham to walk to the Hospital, the view of the attractive little town unfolded. She saw the remains of a building known as The Castle. Built early in the 12th century as a fortified manor house it has the earliest complete hall of any English castle, with a fireplace in the middle of this beautiful room. She noticed an ancient church (14th century with a show-piece 14th century spire) in the quiet town areas, before she followed the Ashwell Road where the Hospital drive entrance was guarded by two yew trees. The road led to the village of Ashwell where there was an open prison whose trained choir enriched the Hospital social life.

In this county of Rutland rural life was cohesive and amongst the field sports hunting was still active. The Hospital, formerly known as the Rutland and Stamford Workhouse Institution, had escaped any formal appearance as it had been built in the 1800's in an E-shape on the lines of an Elizabethan mansion. It was no longer linked to Stamford and had reached the end of its useful life.

To supplement the accommodation, a one-storey wooden modern wing had been added for 40 patients. At the end of Mary's nine years at Catmose these were the only fully resident places remaining, as the old building deteriorated. Initially there were just under 100 patients (the crucial number above which staff salaries were upgraded).

There was a pleasant house for Matron with two nice bedrooms, a bathroom, sitting room, dining room and kitchen. This was Crown property so its lack of a back door, which terrified the fire brigade, failed to condemn it.

Here, after working a month's notice at Peterborough, Mary brought her furniture and dependent Elise, described by Mary as a "guest dependent." Elise was well enough to do the housekeeping and to enjoy helping the hospital gardener.

Mary now had the administrative freedom to introduce practices in the care of the elderly which in many cases were 30 years in advance of the general outlook. The old building was crumbling but to many residents Mary brought life, mobility and independence enough to go home. In fulfilling her aims she was helped by the supportive social structures of the local community. Here Mary was able to exploit opportunities to expand on earlier experience and to make practical and written contributions to nursing practice in the care of the elderly.

Mary's Educational Aims

She knew that the acceptance of the fruit of her researches would be dependent on education and publicity. She set about achieving this with the same enthusiasm that she gave to the patients in her care. Her earlier professional contacts, her quick perception of an ally, the stimulus given to the positive elements in her staff, made those nine Catmose years the culmination of her nursing work.

Mary died before we could gain from her those illuminating human anecdotes of this period but carefully compiled in neat files, is her professional documentation and news-cuttings.

Amongst the professional documentation is the one personal letter to Elise. By September after the June arrival Mary must have been confident enough in her staff and Elise's mental health to leave Catmose to attend a Personnel Management Course. There she met Beatrice Bedwell, later Mrs. Frank Cooper, who was Matron at the Children's Hospital at Carshalton, Surrey who invited her to stay for a break the following Easter.

Was the letter retained for the happiness it conveys?

Tudor Cottage.

"It is a glorious day. I'm sitting by the open windows with the sun pouring in and wonderfully warm. Murmurs of voices from the next garden blend with the birdsong, and the humming of the bees. The wind gentle, but strong enough to make the trees sigh like the strings of a double bass.

Below, Bea is scraping away at the paint before she starts her glorious sloshing. It isn't wise to be in the vicinity when she starts, everything gets covered."

Mary is entranced by the scene of yellow and white daffodils and wood anenomes across the lush green lawn.

"Leaving the garden into the woods is like entering Paradise. Alone, lost in a few moments within the undergrowth, lured by the bright eyes of the primroses and the nodding purity of the wood anenomes. Careful, here are the modest violets anxious to spread their perfume longing to be loved, but too shy to make their presence known in such heart-breaking profusion of beauty.

"The bunch of primroses and anenomes in one's hand is getting difficult to hold, so stop and look around. 'Whrr'! the woodpecker takes to the air and the sun heightens the gleaming colours of his wing. The waterfowl call to each other. The lake! yes there it is gleaming in the sunshine, its shape so formed to let the reflection of the trees mirrored in its depths form a perfect horse -shoe, leaving the centre clear and bright, a paradise for Narcissus and her beauty.

Here is a peace beyond all understanding........"

Mary strolls on along the winding paths to see lichen covered roofs and the white timbered walls of the cottages.

"A kettle is singing "Come in" and one is drawn into the restful peace of the room with the crackle and perfume of a wood fire. This really is a wonderful place. Bea has one of her retired Ward Sisters here. She is really funny.

"I was awakened about 6.30 this morning with a bang on the door "Matron wants to know can you help her with this"? "This" being the electric kettle, it had boiled dry, I was attempting to push the spring back when she said "Of course you'll be a bit weak having just wakened up." Seeing that even Taylor requires full strength to do it, that remark just took my breath away.

"Bea wants me to help her with some of the painting now... Yesterday the Hospital dental surgeon and his friend came for the day. So lots of garden got dug up and we had a huge bonfire.

"Frank's sister has an adorable kitten and 'peke'! They both took turns sitting on my knee. Yesterday the men brought two spaniels, Bess and Annette, one was black, white and brown. the other liver and white. Adorable creatures.

"Regards to everyone,

"Love to you and Whooskie

Mary "

This was the fund of serenity and security and enjoyment which Mary regarded it was her patients' birthright to share, friendship being the greatest treasure.

If a patient was admitted to Catmose who appeared to have no visitors or connexion with the outside world, Matron arranged for it. In the early 1960's a lady came who had minimal sight. She was Mrs. Dwyer, the widow of a partner in a variety act, two men notable in the entertainment world. It was the time when Jack Warner, the actor, was featuring in the popular police series *The Blue Lamp* on British television. Mary wrote to him to ask if there was anyone who remembered the lady's husband with whom she could make contact. He sent the address of his sisters Elsie and Doris Waters, famous for their comic interpretation of London's east end characters 'Gert and Daisy.' They wrote to the widow regularly and Mary read the letters to her. Christmas greetings came to Mary even after her patient had died; then from the sister who was herself eventually bereaved. Jack Warner wrote to Mary in 1967 with a cheque for a funeral wreath and thanking her for the wonderful attention Mrs. Dwyer had received "at your hospital."

Mary readily accepted the new applied technology in nursing care and her written accounts of this professionalism might lead one to suspect a 'band-wagon' attitude. But underlying Mary's efforts was the educational aim to eliminate the suffering and apathy and to bring to everyone the life she so abundantly enjoyed herself.

As well as the professional press she used popular media such as the periodical *Woman and Home.* page 216, October 1969 - "How do you keep old people fit?", lectures to Women's Institutes, a quarter hour talk "A new plan for old people" in October 1967, in the series *Indian Summer* on BBC Woman's Hour. Mary emphasised that care must be adapted to the individual. Prescient in most things she thought of the needs of the voluntary home carer, realising that most of the increasing number of the elderly would prefer to stay in their own homes.

Mary had learned in a hard school how to make the press her ally. On the front page of the, *Lincoln, Rutland & Stamford Mercury,* 5th February 1960 there is the heading *KEEP THEM GLAD TO BE ALIVE.* Matron was replying to hospital criticism.

The article below showed that the journalist had to listen to Mary long and meekly. He quotes her "There have been criticisms because some of the chronic sick have been kept out of bed........ we allow our patients to mix as soon as they are up and dressed, and we even have parties from time to time."

Television was the carrot to induce self-help: "Any patient who needs assistance to get them into bed must be in bed before the day-staff go off duty. Those who can put themselves to bed can remain up until 10.30 p.m. to watch T.V. If a patient can't take his shoes off he has to be in bed earlier, if he develops the ability to take his shoes off he can stay up later."

There is a happy front page picture of an 89 year old together with Mr. J. Kane, newly appointed as "Assistant Matron" - only the second appointment of its kind to be made in this country. "Shortly expected at the Catmose Vale Hospital is the establishment of a physiotherapy department."

Further smiling photographs appeared in a June issue: Mr. & Mrs. Large, patients for whose golden wedding an Alice-in-Wonderland party (the cake bore the iced words EAT ME) had been attended by the 61 patients. They gave Mr. & Mrs. Large (Alice) a rousing reception as Matron escorted them into the ward - the beds replaced by decorated tea-tables, Mrs. Large carrying a bouquet of yellow roses.

Ernest John Saxby, aged 95, pining for his wife, also in her 90's, who had been admitted to the hospital, was accepted as a patient too and there was a grand party for their 65th Wedding Anniversary.

Another happy occasion towards the end of Mary's service at Catmose was reported in the *The Leicester Mercury,* 9th June 1967, when the £4,000 day room was opened by Sir Albert Martin chairman of the Sheffield Regional Hospital Board. Mary reported the general improvement from 1959 to 1966 shown by a decreasing number of deaths: 88 down to 30. [This was a general tendency. Ed.]

Nationally this was an era of cheap food and public sector stability. Mary directed resources to health and well-being.

Nurse Training

Nurse training and conditions of service underpinned Mary's notions for improved geriatric care.

When at St. John's Hospital, Peterborough she had initiated, whilst ridding the wards of antiquated routines, the training of student nurses in geriatric care.

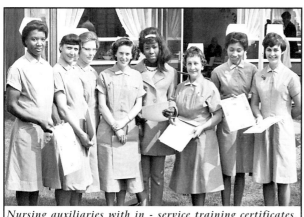

Nursing auxiliaries with in - service training certificates.
Catmose Vale Hospital - 1965.

In the 1960's she had a freer rein. There was a shortage of nursing staff as many other professions were opening to women. They carried domestic burdens too. Mary wrote under the heading "The Successful use of part-time nurses" in the *The Nursing Mirror* 25th August 1961:

"One basic requirement for all staff is undoubtedly satisfactory off-duty. It is nonsense to say that nothing can be altered in the ward. Ask the new student, the nursing auxiliary or even the patients. They are not imbued with hospital tradition and will probably come up with some revolutionary ideas. Try them! If the first ideas do not work they will probably give birth to an idea that will. I have no staffing difficulties, but have a waiting list of people wishing to work in the hospital."

In her implementation of flexi-time, pairing of staff and covering for each other, Mary anticipated the much vaunted "creative company management" of 30 years later. To a secure, brave and intelligent personality it seemed common sense. The photograph of Mary arranging her duty rota braces one for action and service as one looks at it.

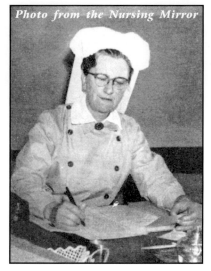

Photo from the Nursing Mirror

Under the sub-heading "Cutting office work" she wrote — "most of it is proof of Parkinson's Law and if nurses refused to do it the great pyramid of hospital administration would be brought down to proper proportions and save the country millions of pounds."

How many future nurses, bound by the requirements of sophisticated drugs and the threat of insurance claims (both embodied in bureaucracy), would like to be such rebels!

In February 1962 the Royal College of Nursing issued a memorandum on the use of part-time nursing staff. Mary had been called in to be one of the working party of 13 Senior nurses, under the chairmanship of Mrs. B. A. Bennett O.B.E., formerly Chief Nursing Officer to the Ministry of Labour.

In another 3 page article in *The Nursing Mirror* 12th January 1962 Mary outlines the qualities of a good specialist Sister.

"The ward sister in a geriatric or chronic sick hospital needs to be a good administrator, a good leader and a good home maker. She must have a wide knowledge of senescence and senility. She must know about public health services, voluntary organisations and all details regarding welfare services. She must be a good teacher, able to convey her knowledge to the patients, relatives and all grades of staff. She must have infinite patience, never be discouraged, be tactful, sympathetic, understanding and firm. She must be a friend to all her patients, but never identify herself with them."

The state enrolled nurse and nursing auxiliaries

Until 1966, Catmose was a component part of the Nurses' Training School of three area hospitals under the Sheffield Board. During the four years from her arrival Mary had galvanised the training course at Catmose and gained a 100% pass rate.

Mary esteemed the state-enrolled nurse (officially recognised only since 1946) highly and used the occasion of the presentation of badges to draw attention to the devotion of the Nursing Auxiliaries as well.

The equipment and nursing methods now being used had made the work easier and more pleasant and the staff had much more time to spend with the patients. In the past 18 months the hospital had been able to send 20 patients back to their homes.

As well as the professional nurse training school Mary organised an In-service Training Scheme for Nursing Auxiliaries. It was a 12 month course, including formal lectures, practical and clinical demonstrations and a 3-week secondment to the Public Health Department.

One of Mary's files bulges with outlines of courses she devised for students, evidence of her effective pressure for care of the elderly to be included both as a component of the official course or as a specialised post-registration diploma.

She approached all hospitals that had introduced different systems of care and must have incorporated or tested many ideas in her own plan of care. The name of Trevor H. Howell, F.R.C.P. Consultant Physician, Queen's Park Hospital, Croydon and Physician Geriatric Research Unit St. John's Hospital, Battersea features much in the pioneer work.

A letter 30th January 1964 from the monthly paper *Nurse* requested readers to submit an article to assist the newly registered nurse in how to train and gain experience in an acute rehabilitation unit or nursing the elderly chronic sick. Mary sent five carefully thought-out pages. Mary herself was a "hands-on" nurse, during the time-consuming fight for the recognition of the needs of the elderly in the wider world.

John C. Best who visited Catmose Vale wrote "Mary used to relieve the ward sisters when they were on holiday so she knew their work and each patient very well." He saw elderly people wanting to live, with lots of stimulation, clean and well groomed, happy and properly cared for and, where ever possible, rehabilitated by staff trained to Mary's high standards.

The staff were encouraged, and were able, to talk about their work and objectives. "I felt Mary was respected by them but I do not think she was close enough to be actively liked. She didn't spend time in an office, if there was work to be done elsewhere."

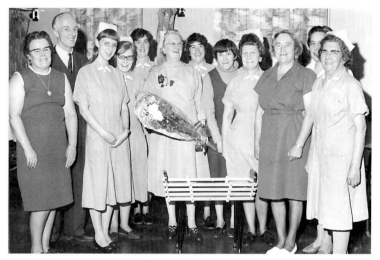

Retirement presentation by the general staff.
Catmose Vale Hospital - September 1968.

Spreading the message: dignity to the end of life. 1962

Mary's vision "to give old people their self-respect and dignity until the end of their lives" was broad, the repercussions intended to be world-wide.

She had first suggested a Geriatric Nurses' Association in 1956 but "It was cold shouldered by the nursing profession" (Mary's words).

A Geriatric Centre

In the late 1950's the big planning and building programmes before regional Hospital Boards were expected to include provision for the geriatric patient. Most facilities were so bad that it was necessary to rebuild.

Realising that the elderly person requires social and spiritual care as well as medical Mary spoke up for a fully co-ordinated service. In July 1961 she forwarded to the Ministry of Health a plan for a Geriatric Centre. The building was planned in such a way as to make it suitable for inclusion in a District General Hospital, or to be self-contained. Costings and sources of income, from meals, rents etc. were included, the Exchequer's input to be supplemented by Local Government and Voluntary Organisations. The plan for a 4 storey building was impressive. Mr. Murray Plester, Dip. Arch. (Oxford), A.R.I.B.A. worked with Mary who typed pages of description. [A synopsis is included in the October 1961 *Hospital & Health Management* p.p. 648-658].

The Ministry of Health really had taken notice. Mr. C. A. Boucher M.B. ; B.Ch. had read about the methods of rehabilitation practised at Catmose Vale and asked to visit.

Correspondence ensued. The Ministry was not prepared to accept the principle of integrating hospital and public health services and a final courteous letter emphasising the unacceptability of providing "Services that tend to mark old people off from the rest of the community."

All the cautious 1960-61 letters from the Ministry are footed by modest signatories and are closely typed on both sides of a small piece of tawny paper reminiscent of war-time scarcity and 15 years later still being used up.

Geriatric Care Association

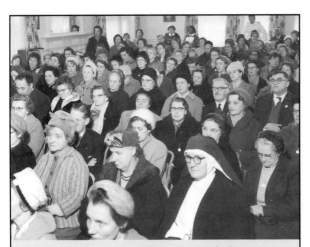

February 1962, St. John's Hospital, Battersea, London. 250 Nurses. The Geriatric Care Association is born. Photo from Nursing Mirror.

Mary outlined her account of the proposed Association. "Much hardship and distress is caused by the gaps which exist between the many services available for elderly people. [In 1995 a 'seamless service'..is still promised. Ed.] It is often difficult to decide whether an elderly person will benefit more from hospital or welfare care. It was comments in the Ministry's letter and my extensive knowledge of Geriatric care that led me once more to propose an Association."

"I met a group of nurses who were interested in my proposals, and consequently the open meeting was called. There was great interest aroused by the advertisement of the meeting and much opposition from the nursing profession."

"It was therefore decided before the meeting took place on 23rd February 1962 to extend membership beyond SRN's and SEN's to registered medical practitioners, the professions supplementary to medicine, welfare officers, matrons and superintendents of nursing homes and those actively engaged in the field of Geriatric Care."

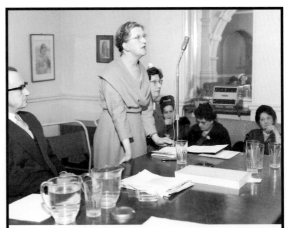

Matron Hodkinson addresses the meeting at St. John's Hospital, Battersea - February 1962

The first Secretary was Miss M. Lyle, Matron of St. John's Hospital, Battersea where the meeting of enthusiasts (and the opposition) was held. It was to be a national educational body. The need for contacts with business and manufacturers was stressed. The first conference was reported in the *Hospital and Social Service Journal,* 7th December 1962. Mary's 3 page article in the *Nursing Mirror*, 12th January 1962 had mustered forces. The first branch of the Geriatric Care Association was, in April, formed in Oakham.

Mary's methods to achieve her aim are best described by one of those talented young folk she quickly identified as receptive fighting fellow spirits. John C. Best, SRN, later Rev. J. C. Best, was at this time Administrative Charge Nurse at Rivermead Hospital, Oxford. His first contact with Mary was at a meeting to discuss the formation of the Association. From a letter 12th September 1995 :-

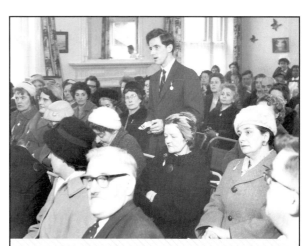

February 1962 - John Best speaks on behalf of nurses who support the idea of Geriatric Care Association, St. John's Hospital, Battersea. Photo from Nursing Mirror.

"I was young and full of ideas but quite surprised to be elevated as Chairman of the provisional committee. Mary was good about introducing me to senior members of the nursing and allied professions and with the then editor of the *Nursing Mirror* also on the committee, I felt I was where the action was. Mary and I would usually have coffee together on the way to meetings when she would float ideas relating to the forthcoming business. She provided many of the items for each agenda and I suspect (retrospectively) that we were all pushed along by her dogged determination and enthusiasm."

"I've wondered what her relationship was with the country's nursing hierarchy and I think they treated her warily and kept their distance — she didn't waste time with fence-sitters."

"She guided me through the maze of officialdom and power structure with advice that has stood me in good stead on many occasions since."

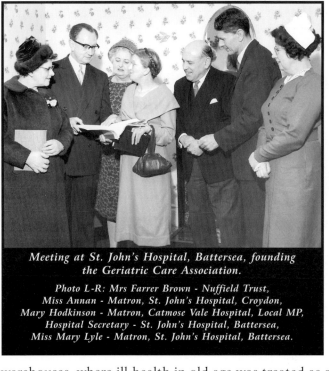

Meeting at St. John's Hospital, Battersea, founding the Geriatric Care Association.

Photo L-R: Mrs Farrer Brown - Nuffield Trust,
Miss Annan - Matron, St. John's Hospital, Croydon,
Mary Hodkinson - Matron, Catmose Vale Hospital, Local MP,
Hospital Secretary - St. John's Hospital, Battersea,
Miss Mary Lyle - Matron, St. John's Hospital, Battersea.

"There must have been a few comments about this unknown trouble-maker from an unknown small hospital in Rutland. She had attacked existing conditions - old people sleeping as many as 60 in a dormitory, no floor coverings, privacy and lavatories far away, by stating "our present hospital buildings for the elderly were never designed to be anything more than human warehouses, where ill-health in old age was treated as a sin and to which it was difficult to attract good staff."

"Here" said John Best "was a cause waiting to become a revolution."

An Exhibition

During a day and evening in September, 1962, with the status of the Rutland, Stamford and Melton Mowbray Branch of the Geriatric Care Association now supporting her, Mary mounted, in the Victoria Hall, Oakham, a Care of the Elderly Exhibition.

The Women's Voluntary Services, The British Red Cross, The Blind Institution and other voluntary organisations put on displays. Ten industrial firms displayed their products - the very latest in nursing aids demonstrated by volunteer patients and nurses from the local chronic sick hospital.

Teas were served by "waitresses" from the Jack and Jill club whose average age was 75 years. Hospital and welfare matrons, doctors. welfare officers, district, student and pupil nurses, councillors and hospital management committee members from a wide area, mingled with the general public of all ages. The exhibition - a feat of organisation - was an overwhelming success.

The aims being educational Mary ensured that it was reported in the *Hospital and Social Service Journal,* 19th October, 1962.

Influence and the printed word

In pursuing her educational aim Mary did not trust merely to correspondence. Her vital little figure must have negotiated miles of city pavements and climbed scores of stairs to offices to see people who she thought might have influence.

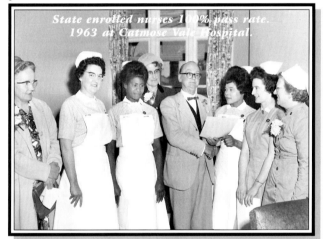

State enrolled nurses 100% pass rate. 1963 at Catmose Vale Hospital.

She had achieved publication in the *Hospital and Social Service Journal.* Now she had more ideas. A letter of the 10th December, 1962 from the editor of this periodical thanks Mary for her recent visit to his office and for her very good ideas which the *Journal* had to put on file "until circumstances change." "You were good enough to put forward a suggestion as to the possible ways in which the *Journal* could help in finding out what those who help elderly people want to know, and answering their queries." *Those who help elderly people!* Again Mary was 30 years before her time: it was on 28th June 1995 that the Carers' Recognition and Services Bill became an Act of Parliament to come into force on 1st April 1996. This was a tremendous achievement brought about by voluntary bodies such as the Carers National Association and hundreds of carers, who over the years lobbied their M.P.'s and Secretary of State for Health. In all her publications Mary thanked voluntary agencies on low budgets, who help carers by listening to them, studying their problems, and finding out WHAT THEY WANT TO KNOW.

A Book

Nursing the Elderly. by Mary A Hodkinson. Pergamon Press, 1966. 154p.

Mary was NOT going to wait "Until circumstances change." Thousands of welfare officers, voluntary carers, home helps as well as professionals, wanted to know how to nurse efficiently. She began to compile a book. She dedicated it to her grandmother, Nancy Clarkson and in her generous acknowledgement she mentions her indebtedness "to Elise Collin, without whose friendship and untiring encouragement this book would never have been written." One can imagine the winter evenings at the typewriter with the usual litter of compilation, having to forgo other pleasurable pursuits in Matron's house behind the hedge, with Elise content as cook and good companion.

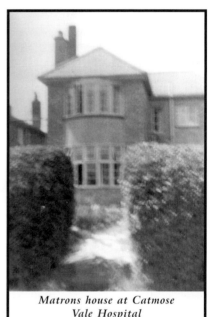

In her Preface she writes "All those who work in the geriatric field derive great joy and happiness from their work." Chapter 1 bears the heading "The satisfaction of caring for the elderly."

"In geriatrics particularly, each patient is unique both in his personality and in the permutations of signs and symptoms he presents. Multiple pathology is especially common in the elderly. These long-term conditions require highly skilled nursing."

Matrons house at Catmose Vale Hospital

The last two chapters cover Rehabilitation and Re-education and Medical and Social needs and services; the last paragraph being Employment - no couch potatoes have room in Mary's world! The professional ease and dryness of Mary's style manifests itself especially in the paragraph on Care of the dying: "It is not essential for his well-being after death, that the patient dies in bed but far too often the patient is put to bed because the nurse believes that his condition is such that he will die fairly soon."

Mary's style is direct, conveying her meaning in short paragraphs and lucid sentences. I believe it owes something to the dignity, clarity and modesty of that of the eminent educator Florence Nightingale herself.

The last chapter on "Medical and social needs and services" as it is written with so much knowledge of the elderly sick person's point of view, is practical in attitude today giving value to the role of the Medical and Social worker and the Chaplain, "close liaison with whom can be of inestimable value to the nurse."

There is an appendix on drugs and equipment. Superseded as it is in many procedures in lifting, care of the mouth, pressure sores - the book yet gives support and encouragement to carers.

After she had submitted her manuscript Mary did not relax. In July 1966 she chaired a weekend symposium held at Stobhill General Hospital, Glasgow. There were six papers by experts on the subject of "Incontinence in old people." The event was sponsored by the Swedish drug company Boehringer Ingelheim Ltd. who funded the 51 page publication of the verbatim report under that same title.

Mary had chosen the subject, aware that it was a disability which most worried the elderly themselves. She introduced the speakers and summed up the whole proceedings, mentioning particularly Dr. S. S. Sutherland who "did deal very clearly not only with the emotional factors of incontinence connected with the patient — but rather turned the tables on us and dealt with the emotional factors as they affect ourselves."

In the 1990's (again 30 years later than Mary) health authorities are realising that "continence advisors", some in special clinics, by their effective advice are obviating both distress and expense .

In January, 1968 (Mary's retirement year) she was asked to contribute to a symposium to be published in the periodical, in hardback textbook form, *Nursing Clinics of North America* Vol. 3 No 4 issue December, 1968.

Letters were exchanged with Helen L. Dietz, Nursing Editor and with Harriet C. Lane, Co-ordinator of the Boston University Council on Gerontology. Mrs. Lane wrote in February:

"The material .... on the Geriatric Association interests me much. My congratulations to you on founding such a practical, much needed multi-disciplinary organisation. We have nothing like it in the U.S."

"...... Corresponding with you makes me more eager than ever to come to England to see your hospital. In your references at the end of your article please be sure to include your own book for it is not sufficiently well publicised in this country."

It was Mary's book that had made her work known to Mrs. Lane. She had written in January:

"Contributors are not paid, (nor am I), but do receive a copy of the book and a generous supply of reprints of their own article."

Mary delivered all that was asked for (pp 675-686). Her photographs of the practical uses of 'chair nursing' (not common in the U.S.) were particularly commended as was her advice on nursing patients with multiple disabilities some needing contradictory regimes.

It was the human complexity of her chosen specialism that fascinated this supreme professional: the older person's "beliefs, attitudes, habits and environment have created a physique and personality all his own." She presented 3 rules for geriatric nursing. Rule 3 is particularly interesting as we shall see how Mary put it in to practice on herself:

" He must be encouraged to live so that his past emotions, experiences and wisdom can be gathered together in the final stage to present a tapestry of a life well lived."

By December, Mary had moved to her cottage in Hoghton. She, who had made hospital a home for so many, had realised that she had none of her own and she must look to her own future in preparation for retirement.

A cottage in Hoghton; The Willows; The Printing Trade

The area immediately across the River Ribble south east of Preston is given its character by the streams flowing into its main tributary, the Darwen. The River Darwen joins the Ribble before the greater river flows through sand marshes beloved of birds, into the Irish Sea.

Hoghton is a wooded region five miles from Preston with undulating pastures on the first rises of the Pennines. It adjoins the village of Brindle which rises further to Denham Hill.

Bells Lane, Hoghton where Mary's sister was living at Miss Thompson's house, is a winding country lane. During a week-end visit Mary inspected at a mile distant a terraced cottage built in the 1860's to accommodate workers at a small power cotton mill. The mill had been sited to exploit the water descending from Duxon Hill nearby and also the proximity of the Lancashire Yorkshire Railway. By 1895 the mill had its own siding.

Ceasing to operate in 1959, most of the mill building was in the 1960's used by a timber firm and clog-shod feet had ceased to pound the dirt road passing the cottage windows which looked out west over a field known as The Butts. The whole area is known as Bournes' after the name of the owner of the mill.

Mary looked at the back of the cottage and saw an attractive garden with a brook at its end and a dirt footpath leading from the terrace row to the mill. There was room to spare for a garage to shelter the Morris 1000 which she had bought from Margaret. The mill stables had been on this spot but now there were no cinders for horse and cart to spread over the pot-holes in the front lane. Soon it was to be tarmac— as two primary schools were to be built on The Butts.

When Mary bought No. 117 the other houses in the two terraces seemed to be owned by members of only four families, demonstrating typical Lancashire social cohension. The mill owner had for £100 sold to occupiers when the mill closed. Next to 117 was a double cottage - it had been the pie and confectionery shop.

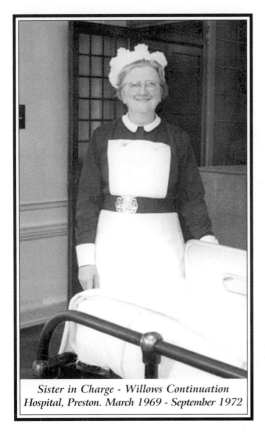

Sister in Charge - Willows Continuation Hospital, Preston. March 1969 - September 1972

The Willows, Ashton, 1968-72

Mary's appointment as Sister at a continuation hospital with less than 30 beds for men, mostly post-surgical from Preston Royal Infirmary, suited her as a winding-down job until pensionable age in a few years' time.

The lovely old house The Willows, in Pedders Lane, Preston (currently used as a Child Development and Family Support Centre) stands on a small curtilage of land conveyed in 1710 to the De Hoghton family of Lancashire from the Hesketh family . It was once the Customs House. Additions were made to it when owned by William Wilding Galloway who was the benefactor who gave it to the Board of Health 1927. This art-loving Lancashire manufacturer spared no expense on interior decoration and appointments.

He employed the well-known garden-architect Thomas H. Mawson. There is a water-colour of the formal garden below a tennis court reproduced from a painting by A.E. Chadwick in Mawson's *The Art and Craft of Garden Making,* 1912.

Mary's working environment was again one of beauty and she enjoyed seeing the patients recover their strength in surroundings, which, in the stringencies of the 1990's, seem luxurious. One could do good nursing there.

A very positive outcome of a bronchial virus Mary suffered in her last year of formal nursing was that she stopped smoking, a habit many nurses acquired during the war, when in some situations cigarettes seemed more plentiful than food.

The Printing Trade

On formal retirement Mary spent the next ten years assisting at Ribbleprint, the Preston business run by her brother. His wife was ailing so he took semi-retirement and handed over to a firm of young printers a sound enterprise which Mary's clerical and administrative experience had helped to stabilise. Harold still acted as consultant.

These were years to enjoy. Elise's health allowed opportunities for excursions and improvements to the cottage. They were able to share many things though Elise was suspicious and jealous of other friends and neighbours who claimed Mary's attention and interest - particularly her sister Margaret. She reached the stage of arthritic disability when she could not negotiate the stairs. The only plumbing was on the ground floor so Mary's carryings and washings must have been reminiscent of the 1940's at Queen's Hospital, Croydon where upper and lower floors shared facilities mid-way on the stone staircase. At the age of 74 years she was a round-the-clock nurse, cook and housekeeper. She knew that she could procure no help other than the attendance allowance which was a financial support.

The mental health of her patient depended on her own. A lively and sociable spirit could not thrive in constricted emotional and intellectual space. Most full time carers will understand Mary's desperation when, in late summer 1985 John Best now living and working in Shetland with his nurse wife "had a phone call from a very distressed Mary asking if she could visit us on Fair Isle. She was exhausted from looking after Elise and had a very painful shoulder and wanted a break in absolute quiet. We were due to go away during the time, so she had about a week with us, then a few days on Mainland, Shetland. We had arranged accommodation there in a lovely bungalow, with beautiful gardens beside a peaceful voe (inlet of the sea), miles from anywhere. Everything seemed perfect - but by this time Mary was feeling better and got the bus into Lerwick every day."

Mary was as totally loyal to Elise as if she were one of her patients. She built on whatever emotional and mental normality remained to Elise. Equality and friendship in the true sense there was not and she confessed to these understanding friends that Elise's now long standing unwillingness to go out of the house, remaining in bed with "Top of the Pops" on T.V. turned up loudly was driving Mary to frenzy.

Elise's personality eludes one. She refused to appear on photographs and Mary's suggestion to "ask my sister Margaret" could bring no illuminating reply other than "I could never break through the jealousy."

The respite enabled a restored Mary to return to duty in Bournes Row, and in her usual way, to turn adverse circumstances on their head. The neighbours too were good to come home to, where cottage doors opened onto the pavement. Mary's friendliness and open manner were well received from her first coming. Sympathetic to all, she remained as she wished to be "Matron" or "Miss Hodkinson" except to a few more intimate acquaintances. One of these said "Mary never made a fuss about anything." She could reassure people about their 'health' with the philosophy "you may have had this for years, now they have put a label on it, it is no different" She took a concerned interest too in the children who played in the lane.

There were only two dramas in this peaceful community occurring within a year or two. Drug dealers and distributors, with concomitant thieving, rented the top end cottage. To deal with a desperate situation, unknown persons concerned for the young "borrowed" a J.C.B. from the timber yard and bull-dozed this house one night. It was a neat job; the nuisance was cleared without many residents knowing about it.

When on an April night in 1991 at 11.0 o'clock the four storey mill used by the timber firm was ablaze no-one could ignore the 8 fire-engines that raced up the lane. The nearby school was open to receive refugees from the nearest cottages but elderly people were standing about at the far end not having heard of this. It was Mary who noticed them and invited them into her house for a hot drink.

The fire was a sad and symbolic end to Brindle Mill where, latterly combing machines had been installed to achieve a silk finish to the fine woven cloth. Here five generations of women had won financial independence and dignity. Imbued with community feeling they and their descendants enriched "Matron's" life.

After Mary died her little "cottage hospice" now empty received daily visits of care from a devoted neighbour.

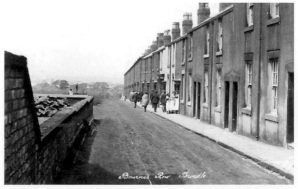

Before the first world war the girls at the pie shop wearing aprons stand near the cottage that became Mary's last home.

Life Long Learning
A room and a telephone at the University, Preston. 1986

Her holiday and Christmas over, Mary phoned Mr. L.J. Soulsby, who worked in Continuing Education at Preston Polytechnic to know more about the informal learning groups for older people being set up.

These baby groups had been born in 1984; in 1986 Jim Soulsby was briefed to foster them. Mr David Lightfooot, Assistant County Librarian was also looking across Lancashire with the vision to develop community use in library space. The Gregson Lane Community Centre, housed at that time the local branch of the County Library and some publicity was launched. Mary mustered 12 to 18 persons and arranged a meeting there attended by Jim Soulsby who put forward the ideas and aims of Life Long Learning. A group was formed meeting at first in members' homes. Soon the little living room at 117 Bournes Row hummed with voices bringing stimulus of ideas and the skills and exchange of a lifetime's experience by these older people.

Elise was to live another year aware in the upstairs room of individual voices below. She died in March 1988 after a short stay in Meadow Bank Nursing Home in Bamber Bridge. The friendly LLL groups particularly support the bereaved in adjusting to a new social situation.

Relieved from nursing, Mary's energy was thrown into the LLL activities but the poor old car collapsed and buying another was beyond Mary's means after the expenses of Elise's illness and funeral.

Each group of Life Long Learning was to be a spontaneous growth. To establish cohesion and a little direction Jim Soulsby steered the miscellaneous and vociferous leaders such as Mary to develop the Life Long Learning Workshops which were held three times a year at the Polytechnic. Groups now spread over a wide range of the North West and, developing from the workshops, a Life Long Learning Forum was instituted meeting twice a year with members attending from the North West area. These were focused on some relevant topic - an outside speaker might provoke thought on sheltered housing, or the Workers Educational Association. Many of the groups became affiliated to the University of the Third Age movement, which had been the origin of Jim's work, together with the then Northern National Organiser Jenny Betts.

Northern U3A Conferences were held in Huddersfield and, Preston (twice each). The Preston events were facilitated by all the regional groups, affiliated or not. The North West Groups contributed much to the national movement, Harold Potts and Stan. LLewellyn both serving on the National Executive Committee.

Because of the ties to the University of Central Lancashire, many of the Life Long Learning groups saw no need to affiliate to a national movement. Gregson Lane was one of these.

A Newsletter had been started in 1984 and posted to leaders of local LLL groups. The Gregson Lane group was, by 1987, well established in varied activities and older groups likewise had something to write about.

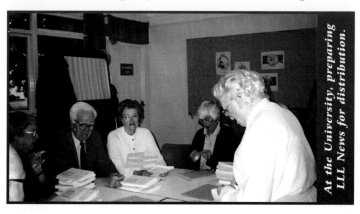

At the University, preparing LLL News for distribution.

Gregson Lane group had developed local history interests and made an attractive wall-chart illustrated by photographs of old farms and homesteads to which pleasant walks had been organised.

Armed with her experience in the printing trade, with the sympathetic, generous pricing of Claughton Press, Bamber Bridge, and with her sister Margaret doing the word-processing, Mary took over the editorship of "News". The circulation of this little quarterly grew to between 500 and 550, reflecting the breadth of outlook and activities of LLL members. Its value in keeping groups in contact is crucial. In 1992 Mrs. Gladys Pilkington having many years before, prior to undertaking a degree course edited the newsletter in its previous form, took over the editorship of the magazine from Mary.

In 1992 awards were made to citizens who took the "opportunity to express their gratitude for Queen Elizabeth 11's 40 years on the throne, through programmes to bring long-lasting benefits." Mary together with Frances Green, Plungington group leader, and others went to the Festival

Hall London to receive the illuminated certificate commemorating the prestigious Royal Anniversary Challenge Award for LLL work.

On the 18th September 1992, the Forum meeting coincided with Mary's 80th birthday , so Mary celebrated this event with her friends from LLL/U3A at the University of Central Lancashire, re-designated from the Lancashire Polytechnic.

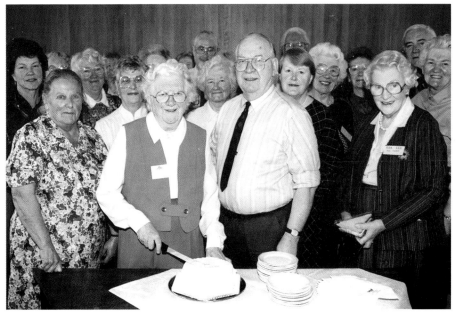

Life Long Learning Forum, 18th September 1992. Mary cuts the cake on her 80th birthday in the company with members of many groups.

1993 ' European Year of Older People and Solidarity between Generations' was recognised by the University conceding, at no charge, the use for a week of the beautiful Arts Centre, the former St. Peter's church, in the centre of the campus. For this Mary took a leading role in the arrangement of meetings, talks, the mounting of exhibitions, including crafts, local history and creative writing, and the securing of publicity.

The following year, popular music of the 1920's was the theme for a day in these inspiring surroundings: "Two men, real jazz enthusiasts entertained during the day and BBC Radio Lancashire joined in the fun."

Mary's enthusiasm drove not only herself but others caught up in something bigger than themselves. She made ripples, which widened their circles even after her death.

In May 1994 Mary made a rare visit to her doctor for medicine to clear a persistent cough. To the amazement of even her doctor cancer was diagnosed. Mary wrote in her notes *Living with Cancer*. "My life had rarely been disrupted by ill health and I accepted the words "terminal and inoperable" with equanimity. My immediate reaction was of Freedom. Now, I was totally in control of my life and I could write the last chapter." The advanced bronchial cancer meant she must anticipate a rapid

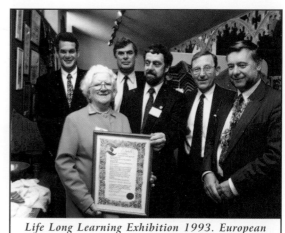

Life Long Learning Exhibition 1993. European Year of the Older Adult. Mary Hodkinson holds the illuminated certificate commemorating the Royal Anniversary Challenge Award.
Philip West of Lancashire Evening Post, Michael Welsh MEP, Jim Soulsby Community Liaison Officer, Brian Booth Rector, Councillor Ken Hudson Mayor of Preston

deterioration within months. Mary filled those remaining nine months with such purposeful rational activity that she altered her friends' attitude to death.

A room and a telephone.

After the diagnosis it took Mary only a month to arrange for tangible benefit to accrue to Life Long Learning in the future. Ever mindful of those not as articulate and confident as she was herself, Mary felt that the busy switchboard at the University and the inevitable wait for the appropriate extension might deter those who had mustered the courage to make an inquiry.

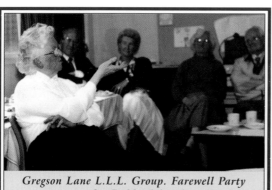

Gregson Lane L.L.L. Group. Farewell Party to the Goddard family.
Mary discussing future activities.
L-R Mary Hodkinson, Len & Marlene Bradley, Margaret Hodkinson & Richard Roberts

A redecorated Council room had been generously allocated by the University for the quarterly meetings, but Mary wanted more. Her loyalty and intelligent perseverance had won the confidence of the Rector in furthering his educational aims of reaching out to mature people in the community. Nearly 400 enrolled students were over 50 years of age. Already the University administered a charitable bequest every two years to be granted to a woman student over 60 to study for a degree.

Discussions for the exclusive use of a telephone for LLL/U3A members were underway when Mary decided that she could make a bequest to "help this along."

The University's response to Mary's intention to leave a donation in her will was itself munificent. David Walsh, Vice Rector of the University wrote in September 1994:

"Dear Mary,

For the avoidance of doubt I set out below those details which we have agreed.

a) The Foster Council Room will be refurbished as soon as possible and this room will be available on a bookable basis to Life Long Learning for use for group meetings, conferences etc. for up to 3 hours per week in one session provided that a reasonable notice period is given for the booking, say one month in advance.

b) The University will donate a suitably worded plaque commemorating your own contribution to life long learning in the University.

c) A small committee room will be furnished and made available for the exclusive use of life long learning. The University will continue to make this room available provided that life long learning movement remains active and the room continues to be used by the life long learning committee. This will be reviewed on an annual basis.

No grinding wheels of bureaucracy here. Mary must herself see as much as possible of what her bequest would promote.

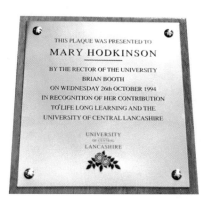

In the simple ceremony on the 26th October 1994 in the Foster Building Council room Mary was presented with a plaque commemorating her work for LLL at the University, together with the keys for room F.61. This handy room off the main foyer was to have its own telephone and office facilities manned by LLL volunteers. Mary's speech gave a resume of the aims and history of LLL; declaring that the gift from the University was an "acknowledgement of the interdependence of all generations."

"In this rapidly changing world it is easy to lose sight of the standards of behaviour which have stood the test of time. May Life Long Learning ever remain a Forum for friendship, flexibility and fun."

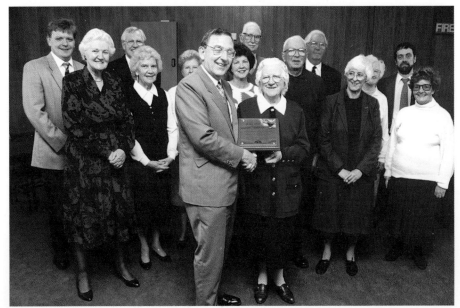

Vice Chancellor Mr Brian G. Booth presents the plaque to Mary.

Tidying up Time 1994-5

During the approaching winter Mary tidied up her affairs.

Early in 1990 she had been asked by a young student for information on the history of nursing. Mary's response was a generous six page script, a copy of which she took to the North Western Area office of the Royal College of Nursing at Graphic House, 18 Fox Street., Preston.

Mary was thanked very positively and encouraged to expand her script for the Archives after it was passed on to the London Office of the R.C.N. and to Miss Angela Gould, Chairman of the History of Nursing Society.

It was decided after a letter to Mary in January 1995 from Susan McGann, Archivist of the R.C.N. at Edinburgh that Mary's collection of papers relating to her nursing career should go there, Lancashire County Record Office being provided with photocopies and details of the location of the originals. She wrote " I am always pleased to receive the papers of an individual nurse as I have found that most nurses do not keep either personal or professional papers. To fill this gap we have started the oral history collection which involves recording interviews with nurses talking about their careers."

The Lancashire Record Office also requested that the government and military documents relating to the family's round the world voyage on troop ships be placed with the Office.

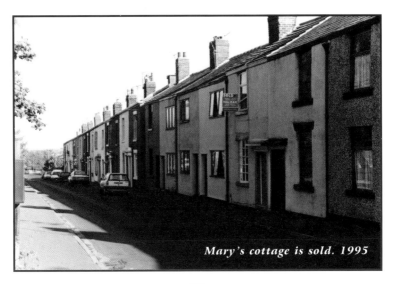

Mary's cottage is sold. 1995

The Life Story

On Monday morning, 21st November 1994 Mary's cheerful voice rang out on the telephone at my Higher Walton home. Would I go to see her to help sort out some papers?

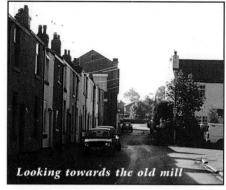

Looking towards the old mill

She had forestalled me, taken the initiative. That very morning I had intended asking her sister Margaret if I might visit Mary. The previous Friday I had noticed at the printer's at Bamber Bridge an attractive card in preparation with a photograph of Mary the text saying "goodbye" to friends. Yes, the master printer, Peter, told me, the end was in sight and Mary was leaving nothing for others to do that she could do for herself.

Within a couple of hours I was at the cottage. She had been told that her life-story was interesting . Would I write it down? The account of the journey across the world made in her childhood was already taking shape. The first chapter owes much to Mrs. Joan Singleton of Ormskirk LLL who helped Mary by listening and typing the result.

Now I listened whilst the clear recollections were carefully uttered. Neither of us made a particular chore of it. Sometimes there was a break in the middle whilst I went to Mintholme Cottage across the railway line to visit Teresa Travis whose writing I had edited and published and which had led Mary to ask me to help with hers. The break gave Mary's throat a rest. I shall always remember with pleasure her smile of approval when I read the tidied script back to her - or was the smile for the recalled enjoyment of her own life?

During these winter afternoons, the light fading across the field through the 'old curiosity shop' window of the cottage, neighbours and visitors came and went. Their eyes focused on the shining spectacles of the little bright eyed lady in immaculate blouse, with neat legs and quick deft movements. Her left arm she began to wear in a sling to control the tremor which the upper chest tumour was causing. But she was still nimble, despite the swelling of the ankles, her easy sociability and warmth of manner disguising whatever discomforts she was experiencing. The visitors smiled as they went, braced by the contact.

Mary had refused medical intervention other than the care of her G.P. Dr. Greening and the comfort the Macmillan nurse provided. With this Sister she had a conspiratorial relationship. Mary wrote to John Best in Fair Isle "I have had two visits from Sister Jenny Garne — and we get on fine — she came with a long questionnaire to fill in. I told her 75% was stupid. On her second visit she had put on the bottom of the form "I AGREE IT IS STUPID." So we are going to write a new one."

A Christmas celebration and a new friend

Mary had allocated funds in her will for a lunch for LLL Gregson Lane members after she was gone. But she decided it would be more pleasant to share it too: the usual Christmas meal she was to book at the Boar's Head, Hoghton was to be her gift, the group not realising this until they tried to pay.

Driving down the bordered Private Road after booking the meal I asked if she would like to call on Teresa Travis at Mintholme cottage. Mary knew Teresa from her *Sexton's Daughter* books and Teresa knew Mary's sister Margaret as the companion of the late Anne Thompson, teacher at St. Joseph's school.

But there was a deeper bond than acquaintance: they met in the serene interior like professionals, the born children's nurse who never had a chance to train and the respected and notable hospital Matron; the eldest daughter of a large family made motherless in 1918 when Teresa was 12, and the Wigan business man's daughter who, after his death in 1917, had taken responsibility for her brother and sister at the age of 5. Each of them loved Brindle and Hoghton and lived simply in a worker's cottage. Mary's cottage was in the terrace to which Teresa's bereaved father had taken his family away from the poignant memories of Chapel Fold at St. Joseph's. Each had been devoted nurses to a sick person in their cottage home.

Their neat becoming clothes and smiling faces, their cheerful, clear voices, each listening to every word of the other, made a duet in the major key, orchestrated with the colour of lives fully lived. It was a special cup of tea we drank, a communion. At the turn of the year Teresa, too, was dead.

St. Catherine's Hospice, Lostock Hall

In early March the woman doctor who had cared for Mary was to leave the practice so there was an agreement that the doctor at St. Catherine's Hospice, established in a former country house and later used as a Continuation Hospital, should assume responsibility.

As early as the late 1950's Mary had attended a course organised for Health Visitors where Cecily Saunders had been asked to introduce the subject "The Care of the Dying". Mary also was asked to give an address. As Matron of a long stay geriatric hospital she had asked to attend the course. For the rest of her career Mary impressed on all concerned the freedom from pain and fulfilment of life - the philosophy of the "Hospice Regime."

Perhaps the movement advocating that the last months of life should be "lived in dignity to the end" was one of the good things that emerged from World War 11: Mary wrote, in 1994, in her notes *Living with Cancer*. "In the early 1950's, just after the introduction of the National Health Service, medical professionals from the Commonwealth and European Freedom Fighters were to be found in London and many International Conferences and courses were held. Many of these senior medical people were amazed at the number of 'Chronic Sick' patients receiving only custodial care and an arbitrary age of 60/65 years was used to pigeon-hole these people as "Geriatrics."

B.W.S. McKenzie, 2nd Baron Amulree (qualified medically in 1936) was probably the first doctor to highlight this situation in a small concise book, easily understandable - *Adding Life to Years* published in 1951. Many forms of cancer were being diagnosed and researched and thanks to this continuing work and the introduction of drug therapy and surgery, were, if taken in the early stages, being cured.

However, the fear of cancer rather than the disease has prevented patients who suffer from the terminal condition from accepting this period of life as the "greatest opportunity to really live."

On her own condition Mary added - "I am virtually free from discomfort and pain and am entirely free to live the remaining months in doing all those things I never had time for in the past."

"The greatest pleasure I have derived from Hospice care is that it is right and I am able to prove it within myself."

On the 10th March fully expecting to come back home after a week's monitoring of her condition Mary despatched her sister (protesting but obedient) on a little holiday she had booked for her, and at St. Catherine's Hospice herself shared a four-bedded room where one woke to the view of the long-established skilfully landscaped garden.

The very experienced nurses recognised a dignified professional who should be addressed by her title unless there was an advance of intimacy. She had specific needs and made them known - one being that she must "sleep in her night spectacles" a life-long habit begun when she must be speedily ready for war-time emergencies. She showed great interest in the nurse's training and self-care in lifting techniques and was alarmed if they put weight on fragile knee-joints.

Mary still had work to do and she ensured that she was dressed and waiting when Jim Soulsby came from the University with the recording machine for her to make her oral contribution for the Royal College of Nursing Archives at Edinburgh.

Impressed as she was by the medical care she was receiving and still feeling keenly responsible for the welfare of her brother and sister after her own death, she wrote a full 3-page record of her brother's present medical situation, hoping that he too could benefit from the best which she perceived he was not receiving. If this was to be a letter, it was not sent, but it was one of Mary's last campaigns for those who needed her.

So the days would have busily passed until her return home. But a blocked lung, and the wonderfully reassuring atmosphere of the Hospice broke Mary's intention to have no medical intervention other than pain relief. At the Royal Preston Hospital every effort was made medically but to no avail, and depleted, she returned to the Hospice.

While nursing Elise and visiting other friends in hospital Mary had acutely observed hospital administration. In 1988 a special full-page report by Tony Skinner appeared in the *Lancashire Evening Post* on the 4th February, after he had interviewed Mary. She had diagnosed the ills of the N.H.S. and expressed a few suggestions for a cure. "There are not enough specialist children's nurses." "There needs to be a revolution in thinking about how nurses are treated — we seem to have got the salary structure the wrong way round — nurses must be paid more."

Her stay in hospital at Preston was Mary's first taste on the receiving end of the new management and of "maximizing the technological through-put" of customers, absolutely outside the control of the patient with minimal communication. She, the fighter for tender nursing care whatever the circumstances could not adjust to this.

She died peacefully on the evening of Monday 27th March 1995. Her brother, sister and friends were there supported by the devoted Hospice nurses.

The light was bright at 11. 0 a.m. on Friday of that same week in the dignified and companionable one-time schoolroom now the Methodist Chapel in Gregson Lane, not far from Mary's cottage. She had arranged the funeral service; but the limited air link from Fair Isle dictated the day.

People gathered quietly. Partly from his own affectionate observation of a working colleague and partly from a final letter Mary had written to him and his wife Betty, Rev. C. John Best, Methodist Minister, Fair Isle. gave tribute to and thanks for the life of his friend and our friend who "felt her life had been planned by a Higher Authority, bestowing to her both the happy wonderful times and the sad or difficult." "Sometimes." Mary wrote "I saw two roads, but circumstances made the choice." "Ideas, actions, people's influence on their surroundings, live on long after the originator's name is completely forgotten."

Characteristically it was her grandmother's rider to the philosophy of Charles Kingsley's, Mrs. Do-unto-others-as-you-would-be-done-by, which burned brightest in Mary's memory. It was " make sure you are the prime mover." Mary's "moves", the enthusiasm she fired people with, ripple on in increasing circles. She wrote at the last "The whole creation of the world, the joys of nature, the amazing building and creation of mankind and the kindness and friendship of people, have sustained my faith in God."

"I only hope that in a small way I have been able to give back a little of the pleasure they have given me - the dignity of service is the ultimate for all."

Early 1995 with a neighbour who visits daily at 117 Bournes Row

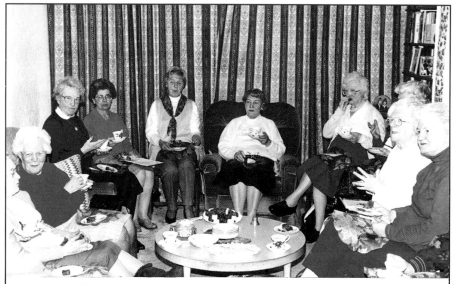

7th Christmas Cake Ceremony. Gregson Lane L.L.L. Group.
9th January 1995 - hosted Stan & Ruth Evans

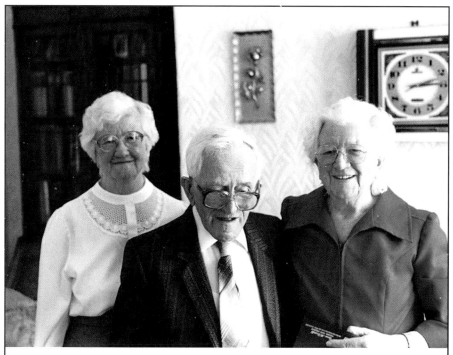

The last family picture at Harold's house in Ashton, Preston

Bibliography

BERRY A. J. *Historical Pageant, Preston Guild 1922.*
George Toulmin & Sons Ltd.

BROWN G. R. *Assured History of the New Church in Accrington 1951.*

ENCYCLOPAEDIA BRITANNICA. *llth Edition.*

HODKINSON Mary A. *Nursing the Elderly. Pergamon Press 1966.*
Incontinence in old people - Proceedings of a Symposium held at
Stobhill Glasgow, 13th July, 1966. Bochringer Inglelheim Ltd.

KUMAR, Chandra & PURI, Mohinder. *Mahatma Gandhi,*
his life & influence. Heinemann 1982.

LIFE LONG LEARNING NEWS. *vols. & 4 1994 & 1995.*

LOG BOOKS. *Deepdale Infants School 1904, Junior School 1904.*

LONGMATE Norman. *The Workhouse. Temple Smith 1914.*

MCKENZIE B.W.S. *2nd Baron Amulree. Adding Life to Years.*
National Council of Social Service. 1951.

MAWSON T. H. *The Art & Craft of Garden Making. 1912.*

PEVSNER N. *Hertfordshire. Penguin 1953.*

PEVSNER N. *Leicestershire and Rutland. Penguin 1953.*

PEVSNER N. & NAIRN I. *Sussex. Penguin 1953.*

PEVSNER N. *West Kent & The Weald. Penguin 1969.*

PRESTON BOROUGH. *School Managers Reports.*
Deepdale Infants & Junior School. 1910. 1911.

PRESTON ROYAL INFIRMARY.
Annual Reports 1928, 1929, 1931.

SNELLGATE Douglas R. *Elderly Housebound.*
White Crescent Press 1963.

STRUTHERS, Charlotte. *Number plays and games for infants.*
Pitman 1912.

WHITE William. *Emanual Swedenborg - His Life and Writings.*
2nd Ed. revised. Simpkin Marshall 1868.

Index

Mary, Mary quite contrary
How does your garden grow
With silver bells and cockle shells
And merry maids all in a row

Traditional English Rhyme

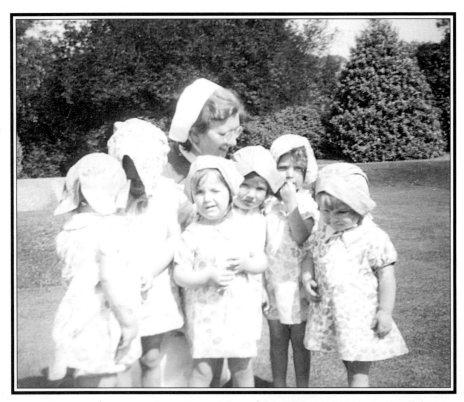

Birmingham children - Burcot Grange, Blackwell, Worcestershire.
Mary - Sister 1937 - 1938